I0765938

Created by <u>Xspurts.com</u>

Get A Free Book At: <u>xspurts.com/posts/free-book-offer</u>

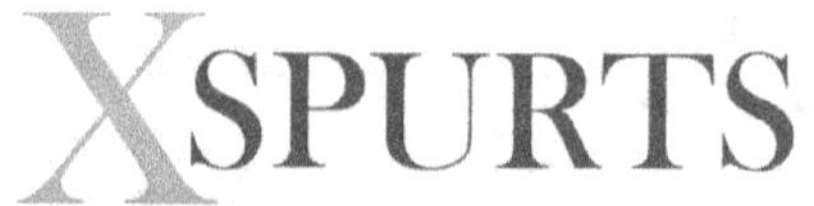

Table of Contents

Table of Contents

Understanding the Basics of Vaping

History and Evolution of Vaping

Different Components of a Vape Device

Understanding Vape Juice (E-liquid)

Types of Vaping Devices

Cig-A-Like Vapes

Vape Pens

Box Mod Kits

Pod Systems

How to Choose Your First Vape

Assessing Your Vaping Needs

Choosing the Right Device

Selecting the Ideal Vape Juice

Setting Up Your Vape

Assembling Components

Understanding Device Settings

Ensuring Safe Usage

How to Refill and Maintain a Vape

Refilling Your Vape Tank

Changing Coils and Cleaning Tanks

Battery Care and Maintenance

Understanding Vape Juice

Ingredients in Vape Juice

VG/PG Ratio Explained

Nicotine Levels and Their Effects

Exploring Flavors of Vape Juice

Popular Vape Juice Flavors

Mixing and Matching Flavors

Customizing Flavors

An Introduction to Vape Coils

Different Types of Coils

Learn to Build Your Own Coils

Re-wick and Dry Burn Your Coils

Advanced Vaping Techniques

Sub-Ohm Vaping

Dripping

Squonking

Adjusting Vape Settings for the Best Experience

Understanding Wattage, Voltage, and Resistance

Temperature Control Vaping

Finding Your Ideal Vape Settings

Vaping Etiquette and Culture

Do's and Don'ts of Vaping

Understanding Vape Culture

Participating in Vape Communities

Troubleshooting Common Vape Issues

Leaking Tank and Burnt Coils

Battery Issues

Vape Device Not Producing Vapor

Health Concerns and Vaping

Risks and Benefits of Vaping

Vaping and Smoking: A Comparison

Addressing Vaping Myths

Vaping Regulations and Laws

Understanding Vaping Regulations and Laws

Have Questions / Comments?

Get Another Book Free

Understanding the Basics of Vaping

Understanding the Basics of Vaping

In recent years, vaping has surged in popularity, becoming a mainstream alternative to traditional smoking. With its myriad of flavors, sleek devices, and promises of harm reduction, it's no wonder why many have turned to vaping. But what exactly is vaping, and how does it work?

At its core, vaping involves the inhalation of vapor produced by an electronic device. Unlike traditional cigarettes, which burn tobacco to create smoke, vaping devices heat a liquid known as e-liquid or vape juice to generate vapor. This liquid typically consists of a combination of propylene glycol, vegetable glycerin, nicotine, and flavorings.

Propylene glycol and vegetable glycerin serve as the base ingredients in e-liquid, providing the vapor that users inhale. These substances are commonly found in many food and pharmaceutical products and are generally recognized as safe by regulatory agencies when used appropriately.

Nicotine, the addictive substance found in tobacco, is optional in e-liquids and comes in various concentrations. s can choose e-liquids with nicotine levels ranging from zero to high concentrations, allowing for a customizable vaping experience. It's important to note that while vaping eliminates many of the harmful chemicals found in cigarette smoke, nicotine itself can still pose health risks, particularly for young people and non-smokers.

Flavorings play a crucial role in vaping's appeal, offering a wide array of tastes ranging from fruity to dessert-like flavors. These flavorings undergo rigorous testing to ensure they meet safety standards for inhalation. However, concerns have been raised about the potential risks associated with certain flavoring chemicals, highlighting the need for further research in this area.

Now that we understand the components of vaping, let's delve into how vaping devices function. There are various types of vaping devices on the market, but they all share some common features.

Most vaping devices consist of a battery, a heating element (usually a coil), a tank or cartridge to hold the e-liquid, and a mouthpiece through which users inhale the vapor. When a user activates the device (typically by pressing a button or inhaling), the battery powers the heating element, which then heats the e-liquid to the point of vaporization.

The vapor is then inhaled through the mouthpiece, delivering the desired flavors and nicotine (if present) to the user.

One of the key attractions of vaping is its versatility. s can choose from a wide range of vaping devices, each offering a different vaping experience. For example, beginner-friendly devices such as vape pens and pod systems are compact, easy to use, and often pre-filled with e-liquid. On the other hand, more advanced users may prefer customizable devices like box mods, which allow for fine-tuning of settings such as wattage and temperature.

Despite its growing popularity, vaping is not without controversy. While many experts agree that vaping is less harmful than smoking traditional cigarettes, the long-term health effects of vaping are still not fully understood. Additionally, the rise in vaping among young people has raised concerns about nicotine addiction and potential gateway effects to smoking.

In conclusion, vaping has emerged as a popular alternative to traditional smoking, offering a wide range of flavors and devices to suit individual preferences. By understanding the basics of vaping, users can make informed choices about their health and well-being. However, it's essential to stay vigilant and informed about emerging research and regulations surrounding vaping to ensure its safe and responsible use.

History and Evolution of Vaping

History and Evolution of Vaping

Vaping, as we know it today, has a rich and intricate history that stretches back several decades. From humble beginnings to a global phenomenon, the evolution of vaping has been shaped by technological advancements, cultural shifts, and public health considerations.

The origins of vaping can be traced back to the 1960s, when Herbert A. Gilbert, an American inventor, filed a patent for the first electronic cigarette. Gilbert's device, which he called a "smokeless non-tobacco cigarette," aimed to provide a safer alternative to traditional smoking by heating flavored air. However, Gilbert's invention never gained widespread popularity due to limited technological capabilities and a lack of public interest at the time.

It wasn't until the early 2000s that vaping began to gain traction as a viable alternative to smoking. Chinese pharmacist Hon Lik is credited with inventing the modern electronic cigarette after his father, a heavy smoker, died of lung cancer. Lik's motivation to create a safer alternative led him to develop the first commercially successful electronic cigarette, which he introduced to the Chinese market in 2003.

The early electronic cigarettes were rudimentary compared to today's sleek and sophisticated devices. They often resembled traditional cigarettes and were powered by small batteries. Despite their simplicity, these devices marked the beginning of a vaping revolution that would soon sweep the globe.

As vaping gained popularity, enthusiasts and entrepreneurs began experimenting with new technologies and designs to improve the vaping experience. One significant development was the introduction of refillable "tank" systems, which allowed users to fill their devices with their choice of e-liquid flavors.

The mid-2010s saw a surge in innovation and diversity within the vaping industry. Manufacturers began producing a wide range of vaping devices, from compact vape pens to powerful box mods capable of producing massive clouds of vapor. This period also saw the rise of "sub-ohm" vaping, a technique that involves using coils with a resistance of less than one ohm to generate larger vapor clouds and enhance flavor intensity.

In addition to technological advancements, vaping culture flourished during this time, with online communities, vape shops, and vaping conventions springing up around the world. Vapers shared tips, tricks, and personal stories, forming a tight-knit community united by their passion for vaping.

However, the rise of vaping also brought about controversy and regulatory scrutiny. Concerns about the potential health risks of vaping, particularly among young people, prompted governments to enact stricter regulations on the sale and marketing of vaping products. In response, the vaping industry faced challenges in navigating an increasingly complex regulatory landscape while continuing to innovate and meet consumer demand.

Despite these challenges, vaping continues to evolve and adapt to changing times. Advances in technology have led to the development of new vaping systems, such as pod mods and nicotine salt e-liquids, which offer a smoother vaping experience and higher nicotine delivery. Additionally, ongoing research into the long-term health effects of vaping aims to provide a clearer understanding of its potential risks and benefits.

In conclusion, the history and evolution of vaping are a testament to human ingenuity and innovation. What began as a simple idea to provide a safer alternative to smoking has evolved into a global industry that continues to push the boundaries of technology and taste. As vaping continues to evolve, it remains essential for users, regulators, and stakeholders to work together to ensure its safe and responsible use.

Different Components of a Vape Device

Different Components of a Vape Device

Vaping devices, with their intricate designs and customizable features, have become increasingly popular among smokers looking to transition to a potentially less harmful alternative. Understanding the various components of a vape device is crucial for both new users and seasoned enthusiasts alike.

At the heart of every vape device is the battery. Vape batteries come in various shapes and sizes, ranging from small, built-in batteries found in vape pens to larger, removable batteries used in advanced mods. These batteries provide the power necessary to heat the coil and vaporize the e-liquid.

Speaking of coils, they are another essential component of a vape device. The coil is a small piece of wire, usually made of kanthal, stainless steel, or nickel, that is wrapped into a coil shape. When electricity from the battery passes through the coil, it heats up, vaporizing the e-liquid soaked into the wicking material. Coils come in different resistances and configurations, allowing users to customize their vaping experience by adjusting factors such as vapor production and flavor intensity.

The tank or cartridge holds the e-liquid and houses the coil. Tanks typically feature a reservoir where the e-liquid is stored and a chamber where the coil is installed. Some tanks have adjustable airflow settings, allowing users to control the amount of air that enters the device and fine-tune their vaping experience. Cartridges, on the other hand, are often pre-filled with e-liquid and are commonly used in pod systems and disposable vape pens.

Another crucial component of a vape device is the mouthpiece. The mouthpiece is the part of the device that users inhale vapor through. It is usually made of plastic, metal, or ceramic and comes in various shapes and sizes. Some mouthpieces are designed to enhance airflow, while others prioritize comfort and aesthetics. Mouthpieces can also be interchangeable, allowing users to personalize their vaping experience further.

In addition to these primary components, many vape devices feature additional features and accessories to enhance functionality and convenience. For example, some devices come equipped with OLED screens that display vital information such as battery life, coil resistance, and wattage settings. Others feature adjustable wattage or temperature control settings, allowing users to fine-tune their vaping experience to their liking.

Maintenance and care are essential aspects of owning a vape device. Regular cleaning and upkeep help ensure optimal performance and longevity. This includes cleaning the tank regularly, replacing coils as needed, and keeping the battery terminals free of dirt and debris.

As with any electronic device, safety should always be a top priority when using a vape device. s should familiarize themselves with basic battery safety practices, such as using the correct charger and avoiding overcharging or overheating the battery. It's also crucial to purchase vape devices and accessories from reputable manufacturers to minimize the risk of malfunctions or defects.

In conclusion, understanding the different components of a vape device is essential for both new and experienced users. From batteries and coils to tanks and mouthpieces, each component plays a vital role in delivering a satisfying vaping experience. By familiarizing themselves with these components and practicing proper maintenance and safety precautions, vapers can enjoy their devices safely and responsibly.

Understanding Vape Juice (E-liquid)

Understanding Vape Juice (E-liquid)

Vape juice, also known as e-liquid, is a crucial component of vaping that plays a central role in delivering flavor and nicotine to users. Understanding the composition and characteristics of vape juice is essential for vapers looking to customize their vaping experience and make informed choices about their health and well-being.

At its core, vape juice is a solution comprised of four main ingredients: propylene glycol (PG), vegetable glycerin (VG), nicotine, and flavorings. These ingredients work together to create the vapor that users inhale when vaping.

Propylene glycol (PG) is a colorless and odorless liquid that serves as the primary base for vape juice. It is commonly used in a variety of food and pharmaceutical products and is recognized as safe by regulatory agencies when used appropriately. PG is valued in vape juice for its ability to carry flavor effectively and produce a throat hit similar to that of traditional cigarettes.

Vegetable glycerin (VG) is another common base ingredient found in vape juice. Like PG, VG is also colorless and odorless but has a slightly sweet taste. VG is thicker and produces denser vapor compared to PG, making it popular among cloud chasers and vapers who prioritize vapor production. Additionally, VG is derived from vegetable oils, making it a suitable option for vapers with allergies or sensitivities to propylene glycol.

Nicotine is an optional ingredient in vape juice and comes in various concentrations ranging from zero to high levels. Nicotine is a stimulant found in tobacco that is responsible for the addictive effects of smoking. Many vapers use vape juice with nicotine as a means of reducing their dependence on traditional cigarettes or satisfying nicotine cravings without the harmful effects of combustion.

Flavorings are what give vape juice its distinct taste and aroma. These flavorings can range from simple fruit and menthol flavors to more complex dessert and beverage-inspired concoctions. Flavorings are typically made from food-grade ingredients and undergo rigorous testing to ensure they meet safety standards for inhalation. However, concerns have been raised about the potential risks associated with certain flavoring chemicals, highlighting the need for further research in this area.

When it comes to selecting vape juice, vapers have a wide range of options to choose from. In addition to considering factors such as flavor and nicotine strength, vapers should also pay attention to the ratio of PG to VG in the vape juice. High PG blends offer a stronger throat hit and more pronounced flavor, while high VG blends produce thicker vapor clouds and smoother inhales.

It's important for vapers to store vape juice properly to maintain its quality and potency. Vape juice should be kept away from direct sunlight and extreme temperatures, as exposure to heat and light can degrade the flavor and nicotine content over time. Additionally, vapers should always check the expiration date on vape juice bottles and discard any expired or spoiled products.

In conclusion, vape juice is a fundamental component of vaping that allows users to enjoy a wide range of flavors and nicotine strengths. By understanding the ingredients and characteristics of vape juice, vapers can make informed choices about their vaping experience and prioritize their health and safety.

Types of Vaping Devices

Types of Vaping Devices

Vaping has become a diverse and dynamic industry, offering a wide array of devices to suit every vaper's preferences and needs. From compact vape pens to powerful box mods, understanding the different types of vaping devices is essential for both beginners and experienced users alike.

One of the most common types of vaping devices is the vape pen. Vape pens are compact, portable devices that typically consist of a battery, a tank or cartridge for e-liquid, and a mouthpiece. They are often designed to resemble traditional cigarettes, making them a popular choice for beginners looking to make the switch from smoking to vaping. Vape pens are user-friendly, easy to refill, and come in a variety of styles and designs to suit individual tastes.

Pod systems have also gained popularity in recent years, offering a convenient and hassle-free vaping experience. Pod systems consist of a small, pod-shaped cartridge that contains the e-liquid and a battery-powered device. Pod systems are often pre-filled with e-liquid and feature a simple plug-and-play design, making them ideal for vapers who prioritize convenience and ease of use. Additionally, pod systems are typically draw-activated, meaning they are activated when the user inhales from the mouthpiece, eliminating the need for a fire button.

For vapers looking for more customization and control over their vaping experience, box mods are an excellent option. Box mods are larger, more powerful devices that offer a wide range of features and settings to fine-tune the vaping experience. They typically feature adjustable wattage or temperature control settings, allowing users to customize factors such as vapor production, flavor intensity, and throat hit. Additionally, box mods often have larger batteries and can accommodate a wider range of tanks and coils, making them versatile options for advanced users.

Sub-ohm vaping has also become increasingly popular among vaping enthusiasts, thanks to its ability to produce large clouds of vapor and intense flavor. Sub-ohm vaping involves using coils with a resistance of less than one ohm, resulting in increased power output and vapor production. Sub-ohm vaping is often associated with advanced devices like box mods and requires a good understanding of battery safety and Ohm's law to ensure a safe vaping experience.

In addition to these primary types of vaping devices, there are also specialty devices designed for specific purposes. For example, mechanical mods are unregulated devices that deliver power directly from the battery to the atomizer without any safety features or regulation. Mechanical mods are popular among experienced vapers who enjoy the simplicity and customization they offer but require a deep understanding of battery safety and Ohm's law to use safely.

Disposable vape pens have also become popular among beginners and casual vapers looking for a hassle-free vaping experience. These single-use devices come pre-filled with e-liquid and are typically discarded once the e-liquid is depleted. Disposable vape pens are convenient and require no maintenance or refilling, making them an excellent option for vapers on the go or those looking to try vaping without committing to a more expensive device.

In conclusion, the world of vaping offers a wide range of devices to suit every vaper's preferences and needs. From compact vape pens to powerful box mods, there is a vaping device out there for everyone. By understanding the different types of vaping devices available, vapers can find the perfect device to enhance their vaping experience and achieve their desired results.

Cig-A-Like Vapes

Cig-A-Like Vapes

Cig-a-like vapes, as the name suggests, are electronic cigarettes designed to mimic the look and feel of traditional tobacco cigarettes. These devices are often the first choice for smokers looking to transition to vaping due to their familiar appearance and ease of use. Understanding the features and benefits of cig-a-like vapes can help smokers make an informed decision about whether these devices are right for them.

Cig-a-like vapes typically consist of two main components: a rechargeable battery and a disposable cartridge or "cartomizer" filled with e-liquid. The battery is housed in a slender casing designed to resemble the size and shape of a traditional cigarette, making cig-a-likes discreet and portable. The cartridge contains a pre-filled e-liquid solution and a built-in atomizer, which heats the liquid and produces vapor when activated.

One of the primary benefits of cig-a-like vapes is their simplicity and ease of use. Unlike more advanced vaping devices, cig-a-likes require no assembly or maintenance—simply attach a pre-filled cartridge to the battery, and you're ready to vape. This makes cig-a-likes an excellent option for beginners or those who prefer a hassle-free vaping experience.

Another advantage of cig-a-like vapes is their similarity to smoking traditional cigarettes. The small size and cylindrical shape of cig-a-likes closely resemble tobacco cigarettes, making them feel familiar and comfortable for smokers making the switch to vaping. Additionally, cig-a-likes typically produce a mouth-to-lung inhale, similar to the sensation of smoking, which can further enhance the transition for smokers.

Cig-a-like vapes are also discreet and convenient, making them ideal for vaping on the go. The compact size of cig-a-likes allows users to carry them in a pocket or purse easily, and their subtle appearance minimizes attention from bystanders. Additionally, many cig-a-like devices feature automatic draw technology, meaning they are activated when the user inhales from the mouthpiece, eliminating the need for a fire button.

However, there are some limitations to consider when using cig-a-like vapes. One drawback is the limited battery life of cig-a-like devices, which may require frequent recharging, particularly for heavy users. Additionally, cig-a-likes typically have smaller e-liquid capacities compared to larger vaping devices, meaning users may need to carry spare cartridges or refill more frequently.

Another consideration is the limited flavor options available for cig-a-like vapes. Most cig-a-like cartridges come pre-filled with a limited selection of flavors, often mimicking traditional tobacco flavors or menthol. While this may be sufficient for some users, those looking for a wider variety of flavors may find cig-a-like devices lacking in this regard.

In conclusion, cig-a-like vapes offer a convenient and familiar option for smokers looking to transition to vaping. With their compact size, simple operation, and similarity to traditional cigarettes, cig-a-likes provide an accessible entry point into the world of vaping for beginners. While they may have some limitations in terms of battery life and flavor options, cig-a-like vapes remain a popular choice for those seeking a hassle-free and discreet vaping experience.

Vape Pens

Vape Pens

Vape pens have emerged as one of the most popular types of vaping devices, offering users a convenient and versatile way to enjoy their favorite e-liquids. These sleek and compact devices have revolutionized the vaping industry, providing a portable and discreet option for vapers on the go. Understanding the features and capabilities of vape pens can help both beginners and experienced users make informed decisions about their vaping experience.

At their core, vape pens consist of three main components: a battery, a tank or cartridge, and a mouthpiece. The battery provides the power necessary to heat the coil and vaporize the e-liquid, while the tank or cartridge holds the e-liquid and houses the coil. The mouthpiece is where users inhale the vapor produced by the device.

One of the key advantages of vape pens is their portability and convenience. Vape pens are typically small and lightweight, making them easy to carry in a pocket or purse. Their discreet design also allows users to vape in public without drawing unwanted attention. Additionally, many vape pens feature a simple one-button operation, making them easy to use even for beginners.

Vape pens come in a variety of styles and designs to suit individual preferences. Some vape pens feature a cylindrical shape similar to a traditional cigarette, while others may have a more modern and streamlined appearance. Many vape pens also come in a range of colors and finishes, allowing users to personalize their device to match their style.

Another advantage of vape pens is their versatility. Most vape pens are compatible with a wide range of e-liquids, including both nicotine-based and nicotine-free options. This allows users to experiment with different flavors and nicotine strengths to find their perfect vaping experience. Additionally, many vape pens feature adjustable airflow settings, allowing users to customize their inhale to suit their preferences.

Vape pens are also known for their affordability, making them an excellent option for vapers on a budget. While some advanced vaping devices can be quite expensive, vape pens are often more accessible to beginners and casual vapers. Many vape pens are available at affordable price points without sacrificing quality or performance.

However, it's essential to consider some potential drawbacks of vape pens as well. One limitation is the relatively small battery capacity of vape pens compared to larger vaping devices like box mods. This means that vape pens may require more frequent recharging, particularly for heavy users. Additionally, the smaller size of vape pens may limit the amount of e-liquid they can hold, requiring users to refill more often.

Another consideration is the limited customization options available for vape pens. While many vape pens feature adjustable airflow settings, they may lack the advanced features found in larger vaping devices like temperature control or wattage adjustment. This may be a drawback for experienced vapers who prefer more control over their vaping experience.

In conclusion, vape pens offer a convenient, portable, and affordable option for vapers looking to enjoy their favorite e-liquids on the go. With their sleek design, ease of use, and versatility, vape pens have become a popular choice for both beginners and experienced users alike. While they may have some limitations compared to larger vaping devices, vape pens remain a convenient and accessible option for vapers of all levels.

Box Mod Kits

Box Mod Kits

Box mod kits represent a significant advancement in the world of vaping, offering users a powerful and customizable vaping experience. These kits, which typically include a box mod device, a tank, coils, and other accessories, have become increasingly popular among vaping enthusiasts seeking enhanced performance and versatility. Understanding the features and benefits of box mod kits can help vapers make informed decisions about their vaping journey.

At the heart of every box mod kit is the box mod device itself. Unlike traditional vape pens or cig-a-like devices, box mods are larger and more powerful, offering users a wide range of features and settings to customize their vaping experience. Box mods typically feature a box-shaped design with a built-in or removable battery, a display screen, and buttons for adjusting settings such as wattage, temperature, and coil resistance.

One of the key advantages of box mod kits is their versatility. Box mods allow users to adjust various settings to tailor their vaping experience to their preferences. For example, users can adjust the wattage or temperature to control the intensity of the vapor and flavor produced by the device. Additionally, many box mods feature advanced safety features such as overheat protection, short-circuit protection, and reverse battery protection, providing users with peace of mind while vaping.

Box mod kits also offer increased battery life compared to smaller vaping devices like vape pens. The larger size of box mods allows for larger batteries, which means users can enjoy longer vaping sessions without needing to recharge as frequently. Additionally, many box mods feature removable batteries, allowing users to carry spare batteries and easily swap them out when needed.

Another advantage of box mod kits is their compatibility with a wide range of tanks and coils. Most box mod kits come with a sub-ohm tank, which is designed to produce large clouds of vapor and intense flavor. However, users can also choose to use their preferred tank and coils with their box mod device, providing greater flexibility and customization options.

Despite their larger size, box mod kits are still portable and convenient for vaping on the go. Many box mod devices feature a compact and ergonomic design that fits comfortably in the hand, making them easy to carry in a pocket or bag. Additionally, box mod kits often come with a variety of accessories, such as carrying cases or lanyards, to further enhance portability and convenience.

However, it's essential to consider some potential drawbacks of box mod kits as well. One limitation is the learning curve associated with using box mod devices, particularly for beginners. The wide range of settings and features available on box mods can be overwhelming for new users, and it may take some time to familiarize oneself with all the functions and capabilities of the device.

Another consideration is the higher cost of box mod kits compared to smaller vaping devices like vape pens. While box mod kits offer increased performance and customization options, they also come with a higher price tag. Additionally, users may need to invest in additional accessories such as batteries, chargers, and replacement coils, adding to the overall cost of ownership.

In conclusion, box mod kits offer vapers a powerful and customizable vaping experience with enhanced performance and versatility. With their wide range of features and settings, box mod kits allow users to tailor their vaping experience to their preferences. While they may have a higher upfront cost and a steeper learning curve, box mod kits remain a popular choice among vaping enthusiasts seeking the ultimate vaping experience.

Pod Systems

Pod Systems

Pod systems have revolutionized the vaping industry, offering users a compact, portable, and user-friendly alternative to traditional vaping devices. These innovative devices have quickly gained popularity among both beginners and experienced vapers due to their simplicity, convenience, and versatility. Understanding the features and benefits of pod systems can help vapers make informed decisions about their vaping experience.

At the core of every pod system is the pod itself. Pods are small, pre-filled cartridges or tanks that contain e-liquid and a built-in coil or atomizer. Unlike traditional tanks, which require manual refilling and coil replacement, pods are designed to be disposable or refillable, making them incredibly easy to use. This plug-and-play design eliminates the need for messy refills and coil changes, making pod systems ideal for beginners or vapers looking for a hassle-free vaping experience.

One of the key advantages of pod systems is their compact size and portability. Pod systems are typically small and lightweight, making them easy to carry in a pocket or purse. Their discreet design also allows users to vape in public without drawing unwanted attention. Additionally, many pod systems feature draw-activated technology, meaning they are activated when the user inhales from the mouthpiece, eliminating the need for a fire button.

Pod systems are also known for their versatility. Many pod systems are compatible with a wide range of e-liquids, including both nicotine-based and nicotine-free options. This allows users to experiment with different flavors and nicotine strengths to find their perfect vaping experience. Additionally, some pod systems feature adjustable airflow settings, allowing users to customize their inhale to suit their preferences.

Another advantage of pod systems is their affordability. While some advanced vaping devices can be quite expensive, pod systems are often more accessible to beginners and casual vapers. Many pod systems are available at affordable price points without sacrificing quality or performance. Additionally, because pods are disposable or refillable, users can save money by only purchasing replacement pods or e-liquid when needed.

Despite their small size, pod systems still offer a satisfying vaping experience. Many pod systems feature a mouth-to-lung inhale, similar to the sensation of smoking, making them an excellent option for smokers looking to transition to vaping. Additionally, pod systems often produce smooth and flavorful vapor, thanks to their high-quality coils and e-liquid formulations.

However, it's essential to consider some potential drawbacks of pod systems as well. One limitation is the limited battery life of pod devices compared to larger vaping devices like box mods. This means that pod systems may require more frequent recharging, particularly for heavy users. Additionally, some pod systems may have limited flavor options compared to larger vaping devices, as pods are typically pre-filled with a specific flavor or brand of e-liquid.

In conclusion, pod systems offer vapers a convenient, portable, and affordable option for enjoying their favorite e-liquids on the go. With their compact size, user-friendly design, and versatility, pod systems have quickly become a popular choice among vapers of all levels. Whether you're a beginner looking to make the switch from smoking or an experienced vaper seeking a convenient vaping solution, pod systems offer something for everyone.

How to Choose Your First Vape

Choosing your first vape can be an exciting but daunting task, given the myriad of options available in the market today. Whether you're a smoker looking to make the switch to vaping or someone curious about trying vaping for the first time, finding the right vape device is crucial for a satisfying and enjoyable experience. Here are some essential factors to consider when choosing your first vape:

Determine Your Vaping Style:
Before diving into the world of vaping, it's essential to consider your vaping preferences and style. Are you looking for a device that closely resembles smoking traditional cigarettes, or are you interested in experimenting with larger, more powerful devices? Understanding your vaping style will help narrow down your options and guide you towards the right type of vape device.

Consider Nicotine Strength:
If you're a current smoker looking to transition to vaping, choosing the right nicotine strength is crucial for a successful switch. Nicotine levels in e-liquids typically range from zero to high concentrations, allowing users to gradually reduce their nicotine intake over time. As a general guideline, heavier smokers may benefit from higher nicotine strengths, while light smokers or non-smokers may prefer lower nicotine levels or nicotine-free options.

Decide Between Pre-filled or Refillable Devices:
Vape devices come in two main varieties: pre-filled and refillable. Pre-filled devices, such as pod systems and disposable vapes, come pre-filled with e-liquid and are designed for single-use or replacement when empty. Refillable devices, on the other hand, allow users to fill their device with their choice of e-liquid, offering greater flexibility and customization options. Consider your preferences for convenience and customization when deciding between pre-filled and refillable devices.

Assess Battery Life and Portability:
Battery life and portability are essential considerations when choosing a vape device, particularly if you plan to vape on the go. Smaller devices like vape pens and pod systems are typically more portable and discreet but may have shorter battery life compared to larger devices like box mods. Consider your vaping habits and lifestyle to determine the ideal balance between portability and battery life for your needs.

Research Device Features and Functionality:

Take the time to research different vape devices and their features before making a decision. Look for devices with user-friendly interfaces, adjustable settings, and safety features such as overheat protection and short-circuit protection. Additionally, read reviews and seek recommendations from experienced vapers to gain insights into device performance and reliability.

Set a Budget:
Vape devices come in a wide range of price points, so it's essential to set a budget before shopping for your first vape. Consider how much you're willing to invest in your vaping experience and prioritize features and functionality that align with your budget. Remember to factor in the cost of accessories such as e-liquids, coils, and replacement parts when budgeting for your vape device.

Try Before You Buy:
If possible, visit a local vape shop or attend a vaping expo to try out different vape devices before making a purchase. Many vape shops offer sample stations where you can test different flavors and devices to see what works best for you. Trying out different devices firsthand can help you make a more informed decision and ensure that you choose a vape device that meets your needs and preferences.

Choosing your first vape is an important decision that can significantly impact your vaping experience. By considering factors such as vaping style, nicotine strength, device type, battery life, and budget, you can find the perfect vape device to kickstart your vaping journey. Remember to do your research, seek recommendations, and take the time to try out different devices before making a decision. With the right vape device in hand, you'll be well on your way to enjoying a satisfying and enjoyable vaping experience.

Assessing Your Vaping Needs

Assessing Your Vaping Needs

Before delving into the vast world of vaping, it's crucial to take the time to assess your vaping needs thoroughly. With a multitude of devices, flavors, and nicotine strengths available, understanding your preferences and requirements will help you make informed decisions and ultimately enhance your vaping experience. Here are some key factors to consider when assessing your vaping needs:

Smoking Habits:
One of the most significant factors to consider when assessing your vaping needs is your current smoking habits. Are you a heavy smoker, a light smoker, or a non-smoker? Heavy smokers may require higher nicotine strengths in their e-liquids to satisfy cravings, while light smokers or non-smokers may prefer lower nicotine levels or nicotine-free options. Understanding your smoking habits will help you choose the right nicotine strength for your e-liquids.

Vaping Experience:
Consider your level of experience with vaping when assessing your vaping needs. Are you new to vaping, or are you an experienced vaper looking to upgrade your device? Beginners may prefer simpler, more user-friendly devices like vape pens or pod systems, while experienced vapers may be interested in more advanced devices like box mods with customizable settings. Assessing your vaping experience will help you choose a device that aligns with your skill level and preferences.

Device Type:
Vape devices come in various types, each offering unique features and functionalities. Consider factors such as portability, battery life, and customization options when choosing a device type. Smaller devices like vape pens and pod systems are more portable and discreet but may have shorter battery life compared to larger devices like box mods. Assess your vaping habits and lifestyle to determine the ideal device type for your needs.

Flavor Preferences:
Another essential consideration when assessing your vaping needs is your flavor preferences. E-liquids come in a wide range of flavors, from traditional tobacco and menthol to fruity, dessert, and beverage-inspired concoctions. Take the time to explore different flavor options and consider whether you prefer single flavors or complex

blends. Understanding your flavor preferences will help you choose e-liquids that you'll enjoy vaping.

Nicotine Tolerance:
Assessing your nicotine tolerance is crucial for choosing the right nicotine strength in your e-liquids. Heavy smokers may require higher nicotine strengths to satisfy cravings, while light smokers or non-smokers may prefer lower nicotine levels or nicotine-free options. Consider factors such as throat hit, nicotine absorption rate, and desired nicotine intake when choosing a nicotine strength that suits your needs.

Budget:
Setting a budget is an essential step when assessing your vaping needs. Vape devices and accessories come in a wide range of price points, so it's crucial to determine how much you're willing to invest in your vaping experience. Consider factors such as device cost, e-liquid prices, and ongoing maintenance expenses when setting your budget. Remember to prioritize features and functionalities that align with your budget and vaping needs.

Health Considerations:
Finally, consider any health considerations or preferences that may impact your vaping needs. Some vapers may have allergies or sensitivities to certain ingredients in e-liquids, such as propylene glycol (PG) or vegetable glycerin (VG). Others may be concerned about potential health risks associated with vaping and may prefer nicotine-free options or alternative vaping methods. Assessing your health considerations will help you make choices that prioritize your well-being while enjoying vaping.

In conclusion, assessing your vaping needs is a crucial step in finding the perfect vaping setup that suits your preferences and lifestyle. By considering factors such as smoking habits, vaping experience, device type, flavor preferences, nicotine tolerance, budget, and health considerations, you can make informed decisions that enhance your vaping experience. Remember to explore different options, seek recommendations, and experiment with various devices and flavors to find what works best for you. With the right vaping setup tailored to your needs, you'll be well on your way to enjoying a satisfying and enjoyable vaping experience.

Choosing the Right Device

Choosing the Right Device

Selecting the right vaping device is a crucial step in your vaping journey, as it can significantly impact your overall experience and satisfaction. With a vast array of devices available in the market, each offering unique features and functionalities, finding the perfect device to suit your needs and preferences requires careful consideration. Here are some essential factors to keep in mind when choosing the right vaping device for you:

Determine Your Vaping Style:
Before exploring the various vaping devices available, take some time to determine your vaping style and preferences. Are you looking for a device that closely resembles smoking traditional cigarettes, or are you interested in experimenting with larger, more powerful devices? Understanding your vaping style will help narrow down your options and guide you towards the right type of device.

Consider Device Type:
Vaping devices come in several types, each catering to different vaping styles and preferences. Common types of devices include vape pens, pod systems, box mods, and mechanical mods. Vape pens are compact and user-friendly, making them ideal for beginners or casual vapers. Pod systems offer convenience and portability, while box mods provide advanced features and customization options. Mechanical mods are unregulated devices designed for experienced users seeking maximum customization and performance.

Assess Battery Life and Portability:
Battery life and portability are essential considerations when choosing a vaping device, particularly if you plan to vape on the go. Smaller devices like vape pens and pod systems are more portable and discreet but may have shorter battery life compared to larger devices like box mods. Consider your vaping habits and lifestyle to determine the ideal balance between portability and battery life for your needs.

Evaluate Features and Functionality:
When choosing a vaping device, consider the features and functionality that are important to you. Look for devices with user-friendly interfaces, adjustable settings, and safety features such as overheat protection and short-circuit protection. Some devices also offer additional features like temperature control, variable wattage, and customizable airflow.

Assess your vaping preferences and priorities to find a device that offers the features you desire.

Set a Budget:
Set a budget before shopping for a vaping device to ensure you find a device that fits your financial constraints. Vaping devices come in a wide range of price points, so it's essential to determine how much you're willing to spend. Consider factors such as device cost, e-liquid prices, and ongoing maintenance expenses when setting your budget. Remember that higher-priced devices may offer more features and customization options but may not be necessary for all users.

Read Reviews and Seek Recommendations:
Before making a purchase, take the time to read reviews and seek recommendations from experienced vapers. Online forums, social media groups, and vape shops are excellent resources for gathering information and insights from other vapers. Pay attention to user feedback, reliability, and performance when researching different vaping devices. Additionally, don't hesitate to ask for recommendations from friends or family members who vape.

Try Before You Buy:
If possible, visit a local vape shop or attend a vaping expo to try out different devices before making a purchase. Many vape shops offer sample stations where you can test different devices and flavors to see what works best for you. Trying out different devices firsthand can help you make a more informed decision and ensure that you choose a device that meets your needs and preferences.

In conclusion, choosing the right vaping device requires careful consideration of factors such as vaping style, device type, battery life, features and functionality, budget, and user feedback. By assessing your preferences and priorities and conducting thorough research, you can find the perfect vaping device to enhance your vaping experience. Remember to explore different options, seek recommendations, and try out different devices before making a decision. With the right vaping device tailored to your needs, you'll be well on your way to enjoying a satisfying and enjoyable vaping experience.

Selecting the Ideal Vape Juice

Selecting the Ideal Vape Juice

Choosing the right vape juice is essential for a satisfying and enjoyable vaping experience. With a plethora of flavors, nicotine strengths, and PG/VG ratios available, finding the ideal vape juice to suit your preferences can seem overwhelming. However, by understanding the key factors to consider and exploring different options, you can find the perfect vape juice to enhance your vaping journey.

Flavor Selection:
One of the most exciting aspects of vaping is the wide range of flavors available in vape juices. From traditional tobacco and menthol to fruity, dessert, and beverage-inspired flavors, there's something to suit every palate. When selecting vape juice flavors, consider your personal preferences and taste preferences. Do you prefer sweet, fruity flavors, or do you enjoy the rich, robust taste of tobacco? Experimenting with different flavor options can help you discover your favorites and keep your vaping experience interesting.

Nicotine Strength:
Nicotine strength is another crucial factor to consider when selecting vape juice. Nicotine levels in vape juices typically range from zero to high concentrations, allowing users to choose the level of nicotine that best suits their needs. Heavy smokers may prefer higher nicotine strengths to satisfy cravings, while light smokers or non-smokers may opt for lower nicotine levels or nicotine-free options. It's essential to find the right balance of nicotine strength to ensure a satisfying vaping experience without experiencing nicotine-related side effects.

PG/VG Ratio:
Propylene glycol (PG) and vegetable glycerin (VG) are the two primary components of vape juice, each contributing to the overall vaping experience. PG is responsible for throat hit and flavor intensity, while VG is responsible for vapor production and sweetness. When selecting a vape juice, consider the PG/VG ratio and how it may affect your vaping experience. A higher PG ratio may provide a stronger throat hit and flavor, while a higher VG ratio may produce denser vapor clouds and a smoother inhale. Experimenting with different PG/VG ratios can help you find the perfect balance for your preferences.

Quality and Safety:

When purchasing vape juice, it's essential to prioritize quality and safety. Look for reputable brands that use high-quality ingredients and adhere to strict manufacturing standards. Avoid purchasing vape juices from unlicensed or unreliable sources, as they may contain harmful additives or contaminants. Additionally, be wary of vape juices that are significantly cheaper than others, as they may be of inferior quality. Choosing vape juices from trusted brands ensures a safe and enjoyable vaping experience.

Consider Allergies and Sensitivities:
It's essential to consider any allergies or sensitivities you may have when selecting vape juice. Some people may be allergic to ingredients commonly found in vape juice, such as propylene glycol or certain flavorings. If you have any known allergies or sensitivities, be sure to read the ingredient list carefully and choose vape juices that are free from allergens. Additionally, if you experience any adverse reactions while vaping, discontinue use immediately and consult a healthcare professional.

Experiment and Explore:
Ultimately, finding the ideal vape juice is a process of experimentation and exploration. Don't be afraid to try new flavors, nicotine strengths, and PG/VG ratios to find what works best for you. Visit local vape shops and attend vaping expos to sample different vape juices and gather recommendations from experienced vapers. By exploring different options and keeping an open mind, you can discover unique and enjoyable vape juices that enhance your vaping experience.

In conclusion, selecting the ideal vape juice is an essential aspect of vaping that can significantly impact your overall enjoyment and satisfaction. By considering factors such as flavor selection, nicotine strength, PG/VG ratio, quality and safety, allergies and sensitivities, and experimentation, you can find the perfect vape juice to suit your preferences and enhance your vaping journey. Remember to explore different options, gather recommendations, and prioritize quality and safety when selecting vape juice. With the right vape juice in hand, you'll be well on your way to enjoying a satisfying and enjoyable vaping experience.

Setting Up Your Vape

Setting Up Your Vape

Setting up your vape device for the first time can be an exciting and rewarding experience, but it's essential to take the time to do it correctly to ensure a smooth and enjoyable vaping journey. Whether you're new to vaping or upgrading to a new device, understanding the steps involved in setting up your vape is crucial. Here's a comprehensive guide to help you set up your vape device properly:

Charge Your Battery:
Before using your vape device, it's essential to ensure that the battery is fully charged. Most vape devices come with built-in rechargeable batteries that require charging before the initial use. Connect your vape device to the charger provided or a compatible USB charging cable and plug it into a power source. Allow the battery to charge fully before unplugging it and proceeding to the next steps.

Prime Your Coil:
If your vape device uses replaceable coils, it's crucial to prime the coil before use to prevent dry hits and extend the life of the coil. To prime your coil, apply a few drops of e-liquid directly onto the exposed cotton wicking material in the coil. Allow the e-liquid to saturate the cotton thoroughly, ensuring that it is fully absorbed. This process helps prevent the cotton from burning when the coil is heated for the first time.

Fill Your Tank:
Next, fill your vape tank with your chosen e-liquid. Unscrew the top cap or bottom base of the tank to access the e-liquid reservoir. Carefully pour your desired amount of e-liquid into the tank, being careful not to overfill it. Avoid getting e-liquid into the central airflow tube to prevent leaking and flooding. Once the tank is filled, securely screw the top cap or bottom base back onto the tank to seal it.

Adjust Your Settings:
Depending on your vape device, you may need to adjust various settings to customize your vaping experience. If your device has adjustable wattage or temperature settings, consult the user manual for guidance on how to adjust these settings to your preferences. Additionally, check the airflow control settings on your device to ensure optimal airflow for your preferred vaping style.

Perform Safety Checks:

Before using your vape device, it's essential to perform some safety checks to ensure everything is in working order. Check the battery connections to ensure they are secure and free of damage or debris. Inspect the coil and tank for any signs of damage or leakage. Test-fire your device briefly to ensure that it heats up properly and produces vapor without any unusual noises or smells.

Prime Your Puff:
Once your vape device is fully set up and safety checks are complete, take a few primer puffs to further saturate the coil with e-liquid and ensure proper wicking. To do this, inhale from the mouthpiece of your device without pressing the fire button. This action draws e-liquid into the coil and prepares it for vaporization.

Start Vaping:
With your vape device fully set up and primed, you're ready to start vaping. Press the fire button on your device while inhaling from the mouthpiece to activate the heating coil and produce vapor. Take slow, steady draws from the mouthpiece, being mindful of your inhale technique and the flavor and vapor production of your device.

In conclusion, setting up your vape device correctly is essential for a smooth and enjoyable vaping experience. By following these steps and taking the time to ensure everything is in working order, you can enjoy flavorful and satisfying vapor with your new device. Remember to refer to the user manual for specific instructions and guidelines for your particular vape device, and don't hesitate to seek assistance from experienced vapers or vape shop staff if you encounter any issues. With proper setup and care, your vape device can provide hours of vaping pleasure.

Assembling Components

Assembling Components

Assembling the components of your vaping device is a crucial step in the process of preparing for a satisfying vaping experience. Whether you're using a simple vape pen or a more advanced box mod kit, properly assembling the components ensures smooth functionality and enjoyable vapor production. Understanding how to assemble the various components of your vape device is essential for both beginners and experienced vapers alike. Here's a comprehensive guide to help you assemble your vaping device with ease:

Attach the Tank:
The tank is the component of your vaping device that holds the e-liquid and houses the coil. To assemble your device, start by attaching the tank to the battery or mod. Depending on the type of device you're using, you may need to screw the tank onto the battery or slide it into place and secure it with magnets or clips. Ensure that the tank is securely attached to the battery or mod to prevent leaking or damage.

Prime the Coil:
Before using a new coil in your tank, it's essential to prime the coil to ensure proper wicking and prevent dry hits. To prime the coil, apply a few drops of e-liquid onto the exposed cotton wicking material in the coil. Allow the e-liquid to soak into the cotton for a few minutes to ensure it is fully saturated. This process helps prevent the coil from burning when it is heated for the first time.

Install the Coil:
Once the coil is primed, install it into the tank by screwing it into the base of the tank. Ensure that the coil is securely seated in the base of the tank to prevent leaking. Depending on the type of tank you're using, you may need to screw the coil into place or simply push it into position. Once installed, double-check to ensure that the coil is properly aligned and seated in the tank.

Fill the Tank:
With the coil installed, it's time to fill the tank with your chosen e-liquid. Unscrew the top cap or bottom base of the tank to access the e-liquid reservoir. Carefully pour your desired amount of e-liquid into the tank, being careful not to overfill it. Avoid getting e-liquid into the central airflow tube to prevent leaking and flooding. Once the tank is filled, securely screw the top cap or bottom base back onto the tank to seal it.

Adjust Settings (If Necessary):
Depending on the type of vaping device you're using, you may need to adjust various settings to customize your vaping experience. Some devices, such as box mods, feature adjustable wattage, temperature, and airflow settings. Consult the user manual for your device to learn how to adjust these settings to your preferences. Experiment with different settings to find the optimal vaping experience for you.

Perform Safety Checks:
Before using your vaping device, it's essential to perform some safety checks to ensure everything is in working order. Check the battery connections to ensure they are secure and free of damage or debris. Inspect the coil and tank for any signs of damage or leakage. Test-fire your device briefly to ensure that it heats up properly and produces vapor without any unusual noises or smells.

Prime Your Puff:
Once your vaping device is fully assembled and safety checks are complete, take a few primer puffs to further saturate the coil with e-liquid and ensure proper wicking. To do this, inhale from the mouthpiece of your device without pressing the fire button. This action draws e-liquid into the coil and prepares it for vaporization.

By following these steps, you can assemble the components of your vaping device with confidence and ensure a smooth and enjoyable vaping experience. Remember to refer to the user manual for your specific device for detailed instructions and guidelines. With proper assembly and care, your vaping device can provide hours of flavorful vapor and satisfaction.

Understanding Device Settings

Understanding Device Settings

Navigating the settings of your vaping device can sometimes feel like deciphering a complex puzzle, especially for beginners or those transitioning to a new device. However, understanding and mastering these settings is crucial for tailoring your vaping experience to your preferences and maximizing the performance of your device. Whether you're using a basic vape pen or a more advanced box mod, knowing how to adjust settings such as wattage, temperature, and airflow can significantly enhance your vaping journey. Here's a comprehensive guide to help you understand and navigate the settings of your vaping device:

Wattage/Voltage Settings:
One of the most common settings found in vaping devices is wattage or voltage control. Wattage (or voltage) settings allow you to adjust the amount of power delivered to the coil, which directly impacts vapor production and flavor intensity. Higher wattage settings typically result in warmer vapor and denser clouds, while lower wattage settings may produce cooler vapor with more pronounced flavor. Experimenting with different wattage settings can help you find the optimal balance for your preferred vaping experience.

Temperature Control:
Some advanced vaping devices feature temperature control settings, which allow you to precisely regulate the temperature of the coil during vaping. Temperature control technology helps prevent dry hits and burnt coils by automatically adjusting power output to maintain a consistent temperature. This feature is particularly useful for vapers who prefer certain coil materials, such as stainless steel, nickel, or titanium, which have specific temperature requirements for optimal performance. When using temperature control settings, be sure to select the appropriate coil material and set the desired temperature according to your preferences.

Airflow Control:
Airflow control settings allow you to adjust the amount of airflow entering the tank or atomizer of your vaping device. Increasing airflow can result in a smoother, cooler inhale, while decreasing airflow can enhance flavor intensity and throat hit. Many vaping devices feature adjustable airflow slots or vents that can be opened or closed to customize your inhale to your liking. Experiment with different airflow settings to find the perfect balance between vapor production, flavor, and throat hit for your preferred vaping style.

Coil Resistance:
Coil resistance refers to the electrical resistance of the coil measured in ohms. Some vaping devices allow you to adjust coil resistance settings to accommodate different coil materials or vaping preferences. Lower coil resistance typically results in higher power output and warmer vapor, while higher coil resistance may produce cooler vapor with longer battery life. Understanding how coil resistance affects your vaping experience can help you fine-tune your device settings for optimal performance.

Preheat Function:
Many modern vaping devices feature a preheat function, which allows you to briefly boost the power output of the device before inhaling. This feature helps reduce ramp-up time and ensures a consistent and immediate vapor production, particularly with larger coils or high-resistance builds. Preheat settings can be adjusted to customize the duration and intensity of the preheat cycle according to your preferences.

Memory Settings:
Some advanced vaping devices offer memory settings, allowing you to save and recall custom presets for different vaping scenarios. This feature is particularly useful for vapers who frequently switch between different e-liquids, coil setups, or vaping styles. By saving your preferred settings in memory slots, you can quickly and easily switch between presets without the need for manual adjustments.

In conclusion, understanding device settings is essential for maximizing the performance and customization options of your vaping device. By familiarizing yourself with settings such as wattage, temperature, airflow, coil resistance, preheat function, and memory settings, you can tailor your vaping experience to your preferences and enjoy a more satisfying and enjoyable vape. Remember to refer to the user manual for your specific device for detailed instructions and guidelines on how to adjust settings properly. With practice and experimentation, you can unlock the full potential of your vaping device and enhance your vaping journey.

Ensuring Safe Usage

Ensuring Safe Usage

Safety should always be a top priority when it comes to vaping. While vaping is generally considered safer than smoking traditional cigarettes, it's essential to understand and follow proper safety practices to minimize risks and ensure a positive vaping experience. Whether you're a beginner or an experienced vaper, here are some crucial tips for ensuring safe usage of your vaping device:

Choose Quality Products:
When it comes to vaping, quality matters. Invest in reputable vaping devices, e-liquids, and accessories from trusted manufacturers. Avoid purchasing cheap or counterfeit products, as they may not meet safety standards and could pose health risks. Look for products that comply with industry regulations and undergo rigorous testing for quality and safety.

Read the Manual:
Before using a new vaping device, take the time to read the user manual thoroughly. Familiarize yourself with the device's features, functions, and safety precautions. Pay attention to recommended usage guidelines, maintenance instructions, and battery safety tips. Understanding how to properly operate your vaping device can help prevent accidents and ensure safe usage.

Use the Right Batteries:
If your vaping device uses rechargeable batteries, it's crucial to use the right batteries and handle them with care. Only use batteries recommended by the manufacturer and never mix different brands or types of batteries. Inspect batteries for any signs of damage, such as tears or dents in the wrapping, and replace them if necessary. Follow proper charging practices, such as using a designated charger and avoiding overcharging or leaving batteries unattended while charging.

Store Batteries Safely:
Proper battery storage is essential for preventing accidents and prolonging battery life. Store batteries in a cool, dry place away from direct sunlight and extreme temperatures. Avoid storing batteries loose in pockets or bags where they can come into contact with metal objects or other batteries, which could cause short circuits or overheating. Consider using a battery case or holder to keep batteries organized and protected when not in use.

Handle E-Liquids with Care:
E-liquids contain various ingredients, including nicotine, flavorings, and base liquids such as propylene glycol (PG) and vegetable glycerin (VG). Handle e-liquids with care and keep them out of reach of children and pets. Always store e-liquids in child-resistant containers and avoid exposing them to heat or sunlight, which can degrade the quality of the ingredients. In case of accidental exposure to e-liquid, wash skin thoroughly with soap and water and seek medical attention if necessary.

Monitor Device Performance:
Pay attention to how your vaping device performs and be on the lookout for any signs of malfunction or damage. If you notice unusual noises, leaks, or overheating, stop using the device immediately and inspect it for any issues. Regularly clean and maintain your vaping device according to the manufacturer's recommendations to ensure optimal performance and safety.

Practice Proper Vaping Etiquette:
When vaping in public or around others, be considerate of those around you and practice proper vaping etiquette. Avoid vaping in confined spaces where others may be sensitive to vapor, such as public transportation, restaurants, or crowded areas. Respect designated vaping areas and follow any local regulations or restrictions regarding vaping in public places.

Educate Yourself:
Stay informed about vaping-related topics, including safety practices, regulations, and emerging research. Keep up to date with reputable sources of information and seek guidance from experienced vapers or vaping community forums. By educating yourself about vaping safety, you can make informed decisions and help promote responsible vaping practices.

In conclusion, ensuring safe usage of your vaping device is essential for protecting your health and well-being. By following these tips and adopting responsible vaping practices, you can minimize risks and enjoy a positive vaping experience. Remember to prioritize quality products, read the user manual, handle batteries and e-liquids with care, monitor device performance, practice proper vaping etiquette, and stay informed about vaping safety. With vigilance and caution, you can vape safely and responsibly for years to come.

How to Refill and Maintain a Vape

How to Refill and Maintain a Vape

Refilling and maintaining your vape device is essential for ensuring a consistent and enjoyable vaping experience. Whether you're using a simple vape pen or a more advanced box mod, proper maintenance helps prolong the life of your device and enhances the flavor and vapor production of your e-liquids. Here's a comprehensive guide on how to refill and maintain your vape device:

Refilling Your Tank:
Refilling your vape tank with e-liquid is a straightforward process, but it's essential to do it correctly to avoid spills and leaks. Follow these steps to refill your tank safely and efficiently:

Unscrew the top cap or bottom base of your tank to access the e-liquid reservoir.
Hold the tank at a slight angle and carefully pour your chosen e-liquid into the tank, being mindful not to overfill it.
Avoid getting e-liquid into the central airflow tube, as this can cause leaking and flooding.
Once the tank is filled to your desired level, securely screw the top cap or bottom base back onto the tank to seal it.
Prime Your Coil:
Before using a new coil or refilling your tank with e-liquid, it's essential to prime the coil to ensure proper wicking and prevent dry hits. Follow these steps to prime your coil effectively:

Apply a few drops of e-liquid directly onto the exposed cotton wicking material in the coil.
Allow the e-liquid to soak into the cotton for a few minutes to ensure it is fully saturated. This process helps prevent the coil from burning when it is heated for the first time.
Maintain Your Coil:
Regular coil maintenance is crucial for preserving the flavor and vapor production of your vape device. Follow these tips to maintain your coil and prolong its lifespan:

Clean your coil regularly by removing it from the tank and rinsing it under warm water.
Gently brush away any debris or residue using a soft-bristled brush or toothbrush.
Allow the coil to air dry completely before reinstalling it in the tank and refilling with e-liquid.

Replace your coil when you notice a decline in flavor or vapor production, typically every 1-2 weeks or as needed.

Clean Your Tank:

Keeping your vape tank clean is essential for preventing buildup of e-liquid residue and maintaining optimal performance. Follow these steps to clean your tank effectively:

Disassemble your tank by removing the top cap, glass tube, and coil.

Rinse all components thoroughly under warm water to remove any e-liquid residue.

Use a mild detergent or dish soap to clean stubborn residue, then rinse again with warm water.

Allow all components to air dry completely before reassembling the tank and refilling with e-liquid.

Store Your Vape Properly:

Proper storage of your vape device is essential for protecting it from damage and maintaining its performance. Follow these tips to store your vape properly:

Store your vape device in a cool, dry place away from direct sunlight and extreme temperatures.

Avoid storing your device loose in pockets or bags where it can come into contact with metal objects or other items.

Consider using a designated storage case or pouch to keep your vape device organized and protected when not in use.

By following these tips for refilling and maintaining your vape device, you can ensure a consistent and enjoyable vaping experience. Remember to prime your coil before use, clean your tank regularly, and store your device properly to prolong its lifespan and optimize performance. With proper maintenance, your vape device can provide hours of flavorful vapor and satisfaction.

Refilling Your Vape Tank

Refilling Your Vape Tank

Refilling your vape tank is a routine task that every vaper needs to master to ensure a continuous and enjoyable vaping experience. Whether you're a beginner or an experienced vaper, understanding the proper techniques for refilling your vape tank can make a significant difference in the quality of your vaping sessions. Here's a comprehensive guide on how to refill your vape tank effectively:

Gather Your Supplies:
Before you begin, gather all the necessary supplies for refilling your vape tank. You'll need your vape device, a bottle of your preferred e-liquid, and a clean cloth or paper towel for any potential spills. Make sure your hands are clean to avoid contaminating the e-liquid or tank with dirt or bacteria.

Prepare Your Tank:
Before refilling your vape tank, it's essential to prepare it properly. Start by disassembling your tank according to the manufacturer's instructions. This typically involves unscrewing the top cap or bottom base of the tank to access the e-liquid reservoir. Take care not to lose any small components, such as O-rings or seals, during disassembly.

Empty the Tank (If Necessary):
If there is still e-liquid in your tank from a previous filling, you may need to empty it before refilling. You can either vape the remaining e-liquid until the tank is empty or carefully pour it back into its original bottle. Make sure to dispose of any leftover e-liquid properly, following local regulations and guidelines.

Fill the Tank:
With your tank prepared, it's time to fill it with fresh e-liquid. Hold the tank at a slight angle to prevent spills and carefully pour your chosen e-liquid into the tank. Take care not to overfill the tank, as this can lead to leaking and flooding. Leave a small space at the top of the tank to allow for airflow and expansion of the e-liquid.

Avoid the Central Airflow Tube:
When filling your vape tank, it's crucial to avoid getting e-liquid into the central airflow tube. This tube is responsible for drawing air into the tank to create vapor, and any e-liquid that enters it can cause leaking and flooding. Take your time and pour the e-liquid slowly and carefully to ensure it goes directly into the tank reservoir.

Reassemble Your Tank:
Once the tank is filled with e-liquid, securely screw the top cap or bottom base back onto the tank to seal it. Make sure all components are tightened properly to prevent leaking. Double-check that the tank is assembled correctly and there are no gaps or loose connections.

Clean Up Any Spills:
If you accidentally spill e-liquid during the refilling process, clean it up immediately using a clean cloth or paper towel. Avoid letting e-liquid come into contact with your skin or clothing, as it may contain nicotine and other potentially harmful ingredients. Dispose of any used cleaning materials properly.

Prime Your Coil (If Necessary):
If you've installed a new coil or replaced the existing coil in your tank, it's essential to prime it before vaping. To prime the coil, apply a few drops of e-liquid directly onto the exposed cotton wicking material in the coil. Allow the e-liquid to soak into the cotton for a few minutes before vaping to ensure it is fully saturated.

By following these steps, you can refill your vape tank with ease and confidence, ensuring a consistent and enjoyable vaping experience every time. Remember to take your time and be careful to avoid spills or leaks, and always handle e-liquid and vape devices responsibly. With practice and attention to detail, refilling your vape tank will become second nature, allowing you to focus on the pleasure of vaping.

Changing Coils and Cleaning Tanks

Changing Coils and Cleaning Tanks

Maintaining your vape device involves more than just refilling the e-liquid; it also entails regular coil changes and tank cleaning to ensure optimal performance and flavor. Knowing when and how to change coils and clean tanks is essential for vapers of all levels, from beginners to experienced enthusiasts. Here's a comprehensive guide on how to change coils and clean tanks effectively:

Signs It's Time to Change Your Coil:
Over time, the coil in your vape tank will degrade and lose its ability to produce flavorful vapor. Here are some signs that indicate it's time to change your coil:

Burnt or unpleasant taste: If your vape starts tasting burnt or unpleasant, it's a clear sign that the coil needs to be replaced.
Decreased vapor production: If you notice a significant decrease in vapor production, even after refilling the tank with fresh e-liquid, the coil may be worn out.
Gurgling or flooding: Excessive gurgling or flooding in the tank can indicate that the coil is not functioning properly and needs to be replaced.
Coil discoloration: If you notice darkening or discoloration of the coil, it's a sign of buildup and indicates that it's time for a new coil.
How to Change Your Coil:
Changing the coil in your vape tank is a straightforward process, but it's essential to do it correctly to avoid leaks and ensure proper performance. Follow these steps to change your coil effectively:

Disassemble your vape tank by unscrewing the top cap or bottom base to access the coil.
Remove the old coil by unscrewing it from the base of the tank.
Dispose of the old coil properly, following local regulations for battery and electronic waste disposal.
Install a new coil by screwing it into the base of the tank until it is snug and secure.
Prime the new coil by applying a few drops of e-liquid directly onto the exposed cotton wicking material to saturate it.
Reassemble your vape tank by securely screwing the top cap or bottom base back onto the tank.
How to Clean Your Tank:
Cleaning your vape tank is essential for removing residue and buildup that can affect flavor and performance. Follow these steps to clean your tank effectively:

Disassemble your vape tank by unscrewing the top cap, glass tube, and coil.
Rinse all components thoroughly under warm water to remove any e-liquid residue.
Use a mild detergent or dish soap to clean stubborn residue, then rinse again with warm water.
Allow all components to air dry completely before reassembling the tank and refilling with e-liquid.
Optionally, you can use a cotton swab or brush to clean hard-to-reach areas of the tank, such as the threading or airflow vents.
Maintenance Tips:
To keep your vape tank in top condition, consider the following maintenance tips:

Clean your tank regularly, ideally every time you change the coil or refill the e-liquid.
Avoid using harsh chemicals or abrasive materials when cleaning your tank, as they can damage the tank's finish or components.
Store your vape tank in a cool, dry place away from direct sunlight and extreme temperatures to prevent damage or degradation.
By following these tips for changing coils and cleaning tanks, you can ensure optimal performance and flavor from your vape device. Remember to inspect your coils regularly for signs of wear and clean your tank regularly to maintain its condition. With proper maintenance, your vape device can provide hours of flavorful vapor and satisfaction.

Battery Care and Maintenance

Battery Care and Maintenance

Proper care and maintenance of your vape battery are essential for ensuring safety, longevity, and optimal performance of your vaping device. Whether you're using a built-in battery vape pen or a removable battery mod, understanding how to care for and maintain your batteries is crucial. Here's a comprehensive guide on battery care and maintenance for vapers of all levels:

Choose the Right Battery:
When purchasing batteries for your vaping device, it's essential to choose high-quality, reputable batteries from trusted manufacturers. Look for batteries that are specifically designed for vaping and have the necessary safety features, such as overcharge protection and short circuit protection. Avoid purchasing cheap or counterfeit batteries, as they may not meet safety standards and could pose risks to your safety.

Handle with Care:
Treat your vape batteries with care and respect to prevent damage and ensure safe usage. Avoid dropping or mishandling batteries, as this can cause physical damage and compromise their integrity. Always handle batteries gently and avoid exposing them to extreme temperatures, moisture, or direct sunlight, which can degrade battery performance and lifespan.

Charge Safely:
Proper charging practices are essential for maintaining the safety and longevity of your vape batteries. Use a designated charger that is compatible with your batteries and follow the manufacturer's recommendations for charging voltage and current. Avoid overcharging batteries, as this can lead to overheating and potentially cause damage or failure. Never leave batteries unattended while charging and always remove them from the charger once fully charged.

Monitor Battery Health:
Regularly monitor the health of your vape batteries to ensure they are functioning correctly and safely. Keep an eye out for signs of damage or deterioration, such as tears or dents in the battery wrapping, unusual heating during charging or vaping, or a decrease in battery life. If you notice any abnormalities, stop using the battery immediately and replace it with a new one.

Store Properly:
Proper storage of vape batteries is essential for preventing damage and prolonging their lifespan. Store batteries in a cool, dry place away from direct sunlight and extreme temperatures. Avoid storing batteries loose in pockets or bags where they can come into contact with metal objects or other batteries, which could cause short circuits or overheating. Consider using a designated battery case or holder to keep batteries organized and protected when not in use.

Use Battery Cases:
When transporting spare batteries for your vaping device, always use a battery case to prevent accidental damage or short circuits. Battery cases provide a protective barrier between batteries and other objects, reducing the risk of damage during transportation. Never carry loose batteries in your pocket or bag where they can come into contact with metal objects or other batteries.

Replace When Necessary:
Vape batteries have a limited lifespan and will eventually need to be replaced. If you notice a significant decrease in battery life, performance, or safety, it's time to replace your batteries with new ones. Dispose of old batteries properly, following local regulations for battery and electronic waste disposal.

By following these tips for battery care and maintenance, you can ensure the safety, longevity, and optimal performance of your vape batteries. Remember to handle batteries with care, charge them safely, monitor their health regularly, store them properly, use battery cases when transporting, and replace them when necessary. With proper care and maintenance, your vape batteries can provide reliable power for your vaping device and enhance your vaping experience.

VG/PG Ratio Explained

VG/PG Ratio Explained

The VG/PG ratio is a crucial aspect of vape juice that directly influences the vaping experience. VG (vegetable glycerin) and PG (propylene glycol) are the two primary base liquids used in vape juice, and their ratio determines various factors such as vapor production, throat hit, and flavor intensity. Understanding the VG/PG ratio is essential for vapers to tailor their vaping experience to their preferences. Let's delve into what the VG/PG ratio entails and how it affects your vaping experience:

Vegetable Glycerin (VG):
VG is a thicker, sweeter liquid derived from vegetable oils. It is responsible for producing dense vapor clouds and imparting a smooth, creamy texture to the vapor. VG is known for its:

Vapor Production: VG is the primary contributor to vapor production in vape juice. A higher VG content results in thicker clouds of vapor, making it popular among cloud chasers and enthusiasts who enjoy performing tricks.
Smoothness: VG adds a smooth, velvety texture to the vapor, enhancing the overall mouthfeel of the vaping experience.
Sweetness: VG has a slightly sweet taste, which can influence the overall flavor profile of vape juice.
Propylene Glycol (PG):
PG is a thinner, odorless liquid commonly used as a base in vape juice. It is known for its ability to carry flavor effectively and produce a noticeable throat hit. PG contributes to:

Flavor Intensity: PG enhances the intensity of flavor in vape juice, allowing vapers to experience the full spectrum of flavors.
Throat Hit: PG provides a satisfying throat hit sensation that mimics the feeling of smoking traditional cigarettes. This sensation is particularly appealing to vapers who are transitioning from smoking.
VG/PG Ratios:
The VG/PG ratio refers to the proportion of vegetable glycerin to propylene glycol in vape juice. Common VG/PG ratios include:

70/30 VG/PG: This ratio is favored by cloud chasers and enthusiasts who prioritize dense vapor production. It offers thick, billowy clouds of vapor with a moderate throat hit and slightly muted flavor.

50/50 VG/PG: This balanced ratio provides a harmonious blend of vapor production, throat hit, and flavor intensity. It appeals to a wide range of vapers, from beginners to experienced enthusiasts.

30/70 VG/PG: This ratio is ideal for vapers who prioritize strong throat hit and intense flavor. It offers minimal vapor production but delivers a satisfying throat hit similar to that of traditional cigarettes.

Other ratios, such as 80/20 or 60/40, offer variations in vapor production, throat hit, and flavor intensity to cater to individual preferences.

Tailoring Your Vaping Experience:

Choosing the right VG/PG ratio is essential for tailoring your vaping experience to your preferences. Consider the following factors when selecting a VG/PG ratio:

Vapor Production: If you enjoy producing thick, voluminous clouds of vapor, opt for a higher VG ratio.

Throat Hit: For vapers who crave a strong throat hit similar to that of traditional cigarettes, a higher PG ratio is recommended.

Flavor Intensity: To experience the full intensity of flavor in vape juice, consider a balanced VG/PG ratio or one with a higher PG content.

Experimentation and Personalization:

The beauty of the VG/PG ratio is its versatility and adaptability to individual preferences. Vapers are encouraged to experiment with different ratios to find the perfect balance of vapor production, throat hit, and flavor intensity that suits their tastes. Whether you're a cloud chaser, flavor enthusiast, or throat hit aficionado, there's a VG/PG ratio out there for you.

In conclusion, the VG/PG ratio is a critical aspect of vape juice that significantly impacts the vaping experience. By understanding the characteristics of vegetable glycerin and propylene glycol and how they influence vapor production, throat hit, and flavor intensity, vapers can make informed decisions about the VG/PG ratio that best suits their preferences. Whether you prefer thick clouds of vapor, a satisfying throat hit, or intense flavor, there's a VG/PG ratio that can enhance your vaping experience and elevate your enjoyment of vaping.

Understanding Vape Juice

Understanding Vape Juice

Vape juice, also known as e-liquid or e-juice, is a fundamental component of vaping that provides flavor and nicotine (if desired) to create an enjoyable vaping experience. Whether you're new to vaping or a seasoned enthusiast, understanding vape juice and its various components is essential for making informed decisions about your vaping preferences. Here's a comprehensive guide to help you understand vape juice and its key elements:

Ingredients:
Vape juice typically consists of four primary ingredients:

Propylene Glycol (PG): PG is a clear, odorless liquid that is commonly used as a base in vape juice. It is known for its ability to carry flavor effectively and produce a throat hit similar to that of traditional cigarettes.
Vegetable Glycerin (VG): VG is a thicker, sweeter liquid that is also used as a base in vape juice. It is responsible for producing dense vapor clouds and imparting a smooth, creamy texture to the vapor.
Flavorings: Flavorings are added to vape juice to create a wide variety of tastes and sensations. These flavorings can range from fruit and dessert flavors to menthol and tobacco flavors, allowing vapers to customize their vaping experience according to their preferences.
Nicotine (Optional): Nicotine is an optional ingredient in vape juice and is available in various strengths to suit vapers' preferences. Some vapers choose to use nicotine-free vape juice, while others prefer to include nicotine to satisfy their cravings.
Nicotine Strengths:
Vape juice is available in a range of nicotine strengths to accommodate vapers with different nicotine dependencies and preferences. Nicotine strengths are typically measured in milligrams per milliliter (mg/ml) and can vary from 0mg/ml (nicotine-free) to 50mg/ml or higher for vapers who require a higher concentration of nicotine.

PG/VG Ratio:
The ratio of PG to VG in vape juice can significantly impact the vaping experience. A higher PG ratio (e.g., 50/50 or 60/40 PG/VG) produces a stronger throat hit and more pronounced flavor, while a higher VG ratio (e.g., 70/30 or 80/20 VG/PG) produces thicker vapor clouds and a smoother inhale. Vapers can choose a PG/VG ratio that best suits their preferences for throat hit, flavor intensity, and vapor production.

Flavor Options:
One of the most appealing aspects of vape juice is the wide variety of flavor options available. From traditional tobacco and menthol flavors to fruity, dessert, and beverage-inspired flavors, there is a vape juice flavor to suit virtually every palate. Vapers can experiment with different flavors to find their favorites and enjoy a unique vaping experience with each bottle of vape juice.

Safety Considerations:
When purchasing vape juice, it's essential to buy from reputable manufacturers who adhere to strict quality and safety standards. Avoid purchasing cheap or counterfeit vape juice, as it may contain harmful additives or contaminants that could pose risks to your health. Look for vape juice that is manufactured in a clean, sterile environment and undergoes rigorous testing for purity and quality.

Storage and Handling:
Proper storage and handling of vape juice are crucial for maintaining its quality and flavor. Store vape juice in a cool, dark place away from direct sunlight and extreme temperatures, as heat and light can degrade the ingredients and affect the flavor. Keep vape juice out of reach of children and pets, and always handle it with care to prevent spills or leaks.

In conclusion, understanding vape juice and its various components is essential for enjoying a safe and satisfying vaping experience. By familiarizing yourself with the ingredients, nicotine strengths, PG/VG ratios, flavor options, safety considerations, and proper storage and handling techniques, you can make informed choices about the vape juice you use and enhance your overall vaping experience. Whether you prefer fruity, dessert, menthol, or tobacco flavors, there is a vape juice option to suit your taste preferences and vaping style.

Ingredients in Vape Juice

Ingredients in Vape Juice

Vape juice, also referred to as e-liquid or e-juice, is a crucial element in the world of vaping. It's what gives vapers the flavor and satisfaction they crave while enjoying their vaping devices. But what exactly goes into vape juice? Understanding the ingredients in vape juice is essential for vapers to make informed choices about their vaping experience. Let's take a closer look at the key ingredients found in vape juice:

Propylene Glycol (PG):
Propylene glycol is one of the primary ingredients in vape juice. It is a colorless, odorless liquid that is commonly used in food additives, pharmaceuticals, and personal care products. In vape juice, PG serves several purposes:

Flavor carrier: PG is known for its ability to carry flavor effectively, enhancing the taste of vape juice.
Throat hit: PG contributes to the throat hit sensation that mimics the feeling of smoking traditional cigarettes, making it an essential ingredient for vapers who are transitioning from smoking.
Thin consistency: PG has a relatively thin consistency, which helps vape juice flow easily through the wick and into the coil of the vaping device.
Vegetable Glycerin (VG):
Vegetable glycerin is another primary ingredient in vape juice. It is a clear, viscous liquid that is derived from vegetable oils. In vape juice, VG serves several purposes:

Vapor production: VG is responsible for producing dense vapor clouds when heated by the coil of the vaping device.
Smoothness: VG imparts a smooth, creamy texture to the vapor, enhancing the overall vaping experience.
Sweetness: VG has a slightly sweet taste, which can contribute to the overall flavor profile of vape juice.
Flavorings:
Flavorings are added to vape juice to create a wide variety of tastes and sensations. These flavorings can range from fruit and dessert flavors to menthol and tobacco flavors, allowing vapers to customize their vaping experience according to their preferences. Flavorings are typically food-grade additives that are safe for consumption. However, it's essential to purchase vape juice from reputable manufacturers that use high-quality, FDA-approved flavorings to ensure safety and quality.

Nicotine (Optional):
Nicotine is an optional ingredient in vape juice and is available in various strengths to suit vapers' preferences. Some vapers choose to use nicotine-free vape juice, while others prefer to include nicotine to satisfy their cravings. Nicotine is typically derived from tobacco leaves and is available in concentrations ranging from 0mg/ml (nicotine-free) to 50mg/ml or higher for vapers who require a higher concentration of nicotine. It's crucial for vapers to handle nicotine-containing vape juice with care and keep it out of reach of children and pets.

Water:
Water is sometimes added to vape juice to dilute the ingredients and adjust the viscosity of the liquid. However, water is not typically listed as a primary ingredient in vape juice, as it is often included in small amounts and serves mainly as a carrier for other ingredients.

In conclusion, vape juice is comprised of several key ingredients, including propylene glycol, vegetable glycerin, flavorings, nicotine (optional), and water. Understanding these ingredients and their roles in vape juice is essential for vapers to make informed choices about their vaping experience. By purchasing vape juice from reputable manufacturers that use high-quality ingredients, vapers can enjoy a safe, satisfying, and flavorful vaping experience.

Nicotine Levels and Their Effects

Nicotine Levels and Their Effects

Nicotine is a central component of traditional tobacco products and is also commonly found in vape juice. Vapers have the option to choose vape juice with varying nicotine levels, ranging from nicotine-free to high concentrations. Understanding nicotine levels and their effects is crucial for vapers to make informed decisions about their vaping experience. Let's explore the different nicotine levels available and their effects on the body:

Nicotine Levels:
Nicotine levels in vape juice are typically measured in milligrams per milliliter (mg/ml) and indicate the concentration of nicotine present in the liquid. Common nicotine levels include:

0mg/ml: Nicotine-free vape juice contains no nicotine and is suitable for vapers who wish to enjoy the flavor and sensation of vaping without the addictive properties of nicotine. It's also ideal for vapers who have successfully weaned themselves off nicotine but still enjoy vaping.
3mg/ml: Low nicotine vape juice contains a minimal amount of nicotine and is suitable for vapers who want a mild nicotine hit or are in the process of reducing their nicotine intake.
6mg/ml: Medium nicotine vape juice provides a moderate nicotine hit and is suitable for vapers who prefer a noticeable but not overpowering dose of nicotine.
12mg/ml: High nicotine vape juice delivers a substantial nicotine hit and is suitable for vapers who have a higher nicotine tolerance or are heavy smokers looking to transition to vaping.
18mg/ml or higher: Extra high nicotine vape juice contains a potent dose of nicotine and is recommended for vapers who have a significant nicotine dependency or require a strong nicotine hit to satisfy their cravings.
Effects of Nicotine:
Nicotine is a stimulant that affects the central nervous system and produces various physiological and psychological effects. When consumed through vaping, nicotine can lead to:

Increased Heart Rate: Nicotine stimulates the release of adrenaline, which can cause a temporary increase in heart rate and blood pressure.

Elevated Mood: Nicotine activates the release of dopamine in the brain, leading to feelings of pleasure, euphoria, and increased alertness.

Enhanced Concentration and Focus: Nicotine can improve cognitive function, concentration, and attention span, making it appealing to individuals seeking enhanced mental performance.

Addiction: Nicotine is highly addictive and can lead to physical dependence, withdrawal symptoms, and cravings when not consumed regularly. Regular use of nicotine-containing vape juice can contribute to the development of nicotine dependence and addiction.

Potential Health Risks: While nicotine itself is not considered carcinogenic, it can have adverse health effects, particularly when consumed in high doses or over a prolonged period. Long-term nicotine use has been associated with increased cardiovascular risk, respiratory issues, and potential harm to developing fetuses during pregnancy.

Tailoring Your Nicotine Intake:

Choosing the right nicotine level is essential for tailoring your vaping experience to your preferences and needs. Consider the following factors when selecting a nicotine level:

Nicotine Dependency: If you are a heavy smoker or have a significant nicotine dependency, you may require a higher nicotine level to satisfy your cravings and prevent withdrawal symptoms.

Sensitivity to Nicotine: If you are sensitive to nicotine or experience adverse effects such as dizziness, nausea, or palpitations, consider reducing your nicotine intake or opting for nicotine-free vape juice.

Gradual Reduction: If your goal is to reduce your nicotine intake or quit nicotine altogether, consider gradually reducing your nicotine level over time until you reach your desired level or transition to nicotine-free vape juice.

In conclusion, nicotine levels in vape juice play a significant role in shaping the vaping experience and can have various effects on the body. By understanding the different nicotine levels available and their effects, vapers can make informed decisions about their nicotine intake and tailor their vaping experience to their preferences and needs. Whether you prefer a mild nicotine hit, a potent dose of nicotine, or no nicotine at all, there's a vape juice option available to suit your vaping journey. However, it's essential to use nicotine-containing vape juice responsibly and be mindful of potential health risks associated with nicotine consumption.

Exploring Flavors of Vape Juice

Exploring Flavors of Vape Juice

Vape juice comes in a vast array of flavors, offering vapers an endless opportunity to explore and discover new tastes and sensations. From fruity delights to decadent desserts, the world of vape juice flavors is as diverse as it is delicious. Let's dive into the exciting world of vape juice flavors and uncover the variety of options available to vapers:

Fruity Flavors:
Fruity vape juice flavors are among the most popular choices for vapers due to their refreshing and vibrant profiles. From succulent strawberries and juicy watermelons to tangy citrus fruits and tropical blends, there's a fruity vape juice flavor to suit every palate. Whether you crave the sweetness of ripe berries or the tartness of exotic fruits, fruity vape juice flavors offer a burst of flavor that tantalizes the taste buds and leaves you craving more.

Dessert Flavors:
Indulge your sweet tooth with dessert-inspired vape juice flavors that evoke the irresistible taste of your favorite treats. From creamy custards and decadent chocolates to luscious cakes and buttery pastries, dessert flavors offer a guilt-free way to satisfy your cravings without the calories. Whether you prefer the classic comfort of vanilla bean ice cream or the richness of caramelized crème brûlée, dessert vape juice flavors deliver a delectable experience that is sure to delight your senses.

Menthol and Mint Flavors:
Cool off with menthol and mint vape juice flavors that provide a refreshing blast of icy goodness. Whether you enjoy the crispness of menthol or the invigorating sensation of peppermint, menthol and mint flavors offer a cooling effect that refreshes the palate and invigorates the senses. Perfect for hot summer days or as a palate cleanser between flavors, menthol and mint vape juice flavors provide a refreshing alternative that leaves you feeling cool and revitalized.

Tobacco Flavors:
For vapers who appreciate the familiar taste of traditional tobacco, tobacco-flavored vape juice offers an authentic alternative that satisfies cravings without the smoke. From bold blends reminiscent of fine cigars to smooth varieties inspired by premium pipe tobacco, tobacco flavors provide a rich and robust vaping experience that captures the essence of classic tobacco without the combustion. Whether you're a former smoker or simply enjoy

the flavor of tobacco, tobacco vape juice flavors offer a satisfying option that appeals to connoisseurs and enthusiasts alike.

Beverage Flavors:
Quench your thirst with beverage-inspired vape juice flavors that recreate the taste of your favorite drinks. From refreshing fruit punches and fizzy sodas to creamy milkshakes and decadent coffees, beverage flavors offer a delightful way to enjoy your preferred beverages in vapor form. Whether you're craving the zing of a citrus soda or the warmth of a caramel latte, beverage vape juice flavors provide a satisfying alternative that transports you to your favorite café or soda fountain with every puff.

Unique and Creative Flavors:
For vapers who crave something truly unique and unconventional, there are vape juice flavors that push the boundaries and defy expectations. From savory bacon and tangy pickle to exotic dragon fruit and spicy cinnamon, unique vape juice flavors offer a bold and adventurous vaping experience that challenges the palate and sparks curiosity. Whether you're a daring flavor explorer or simply enjoy trying new things, unique vape juice flavors provide an exciting opportunity to step outside the box and discover something truly extraordinary.

In conclusion, vape juice flavors offer a vast and diverse range of options for vapers to explore and enjoy. Whether you prefer the sweetness of fruity delights, the indulgence of dessert-inspired treats, the refreshment of menthol and mint, the familiarity of tobacco, the nostalgia of your favorite beverages, or the excitement of unique and creative concoctions, there's a vape juice flavor to suit every taste and preference. With so many flavors to choose from, the possibilities are endless, and the adventure is yours to savor.

Popular Vape Juice Flavors

Popular Vape Juice Flavors

Vape juice flavors have become increasingly diverse and innovative, catering to the wide-ranging tastes and preferences of vapers around the world. From classic favorites to trendy new blends, there is no shortage of popular vape juice flavors to explore and enjoy. Let's take a closer look at some of the most sought-after vape juice flavors that have captured the hearts and taste buds of vapers everywhere:

Fruit Punch:
Fruit punch vape juice flavors offer a delightful blend of fruity goodness that tantalizes the palate with a burst of sweetness and tanginess. Combining a medley of ripe fruits such as strawberries, oranges, pineapples, and berries, fruit punch flavors provide a refreshing and invigorating vaping experience that is perfect for summertime or anytime you crave a tropical escape.

Vanilla Custard:
Vanilla custard vape juice flavors are a timeless classic that never goes out of style. With their creamy texture and rich, velvety taste, vanilla custard flavors offer a luxurious indulgence that satisfies the sweet tooth and provides a comforting vaping experience reminiscent of homemade desserts. Perfect for vapers who enjoy the smoothness of vanilla and the richness of custard, vanilla custard flavors are a popular choice for all-day vaping.

Strawberry Kiwi:
Strawberry kiwi vape juice flavors combine the sweetness of ripe strawberries with the tartness of fresh kiwi fruit to create a harmonious blend of flavors that is both refreshing and satisfying. With their bright and fruity profiles, strawberry kiwi flavors offer a burst of summertime goodness that is perfect for vapers looking to add a touch of sweetness to their vaping routine.

Minty Menthol:
Minty menthol vape juice flavors provide a cool and invigorating sensation that refreshes the palate and leaves vapers feeling revitalized. With their crisp and icy profiles, menthol flavors are a popular choice for vapers who enjoy a clean and refreshing vaping experience. Whether you prefer the sharpness of peppermint or the coolness of spearmint, minty menthol flavors offer a refreshing alternative that is perfect for hot summer days or as a palate cleanser between flavors.

Blue Raspberry:
Blue raspberry vape juice flavors offer a bold and tangy taste that is sure to make your mouth water. With their vibrant blue hue and sweet, fruity flavor, blue raspberry flavors provide a fun and playful vaping experience that appeals to vapers of all ages. Whether you're a fan of sour candies or simply enjoy the tartness of raspberries, blue raspberry flavors offer a deliciously satisfying option that is perfect for satisfying your sweet tooth cravings.

Caramel Macchiato:
Caramel macchiato vape juice flavors capture the indulgent taste of your favorite coffeehouse beverage in vapor form. With their rich and creamy profiles, caramel macchiato flavors offer a decadent treat for coffee lovers who enjoy the sweetness of caramel and the richness of espresso. Perfect for mornings, afternoons, or anytime you need a pick-me-up, caramel macchiato flavors provide a luxurious vaping experience that is sure to delight your senses.

Tobacco Blend:
Tobacco blend vape juice flavors offer a familiar and comforting taste that appeals to vapers who appreciate the rich and robust flavor of traditional tobacco. With their smooth and earthy profiles, tobacco blend flavors provide a satisfying alternative to smoking and are perfect for vapers looking to transition away from cigarettes. Whether you prefer the boldness of Virginia tobacco or the smoothness of Cavendish, tobacco blend flavors offer a classic option that never goes out of style.

In conclusion, popular vape juice flavors offer a wide range of options for vapers to explore and enjoy. Whether you prefer the sweetness of fruity delights, the richness of dessert-inspired treats, the refreshment of minty menthol, or the familiarity of tobacco, there's a vape juice flavor to suit every taste and preference. With their diverse and innovative profiles, popular vape juice flavors continue to captivate vapers worldwide and provide endless opportunities for flavor discovery and enjoyment.

Mixing and Matching Flavors

Mixing and Matching Flavors in Vaping

Vaping has evolved into a creative and customizable experience, offering enthusiasts the opportunity to experiment with various flavors and combinations. One of the most exciting aspects of vaping is mixing and matching flavors to create unique and personalized vaping experiences. From fruity concoctions to decadent desserts, the possibilities are endless when it comes to combining vape juice flavors. Let's delve into the art of mixing and matching flavors in vaping and explore how vapers can unleash their creativity to discover new and exciting flavor combinations:

Understanding Flavor Profiles:
Before embarking on your flavor-mixing journey, it's essential to understand the flavor profiles of different vape juice flavors. Vape juice flavors can be categorized into several broad categories, including fruity, dessert, menthol, tobacco, and beverage flavors. Each flavor category offers its unique characteristics and taste profiles, providing vapers with a diverse palette to work with when mixing and matching flavors.

Experimentation and Creativity:
Mixing and matching flavors in vaping is all about experimentation and creativity. Vapers have the freedom to combine different flavors in various proportions to create custom blends that suit their preferences. Whether you're a flavor enthusiast looking to push the boundaries or a novice vaper exploring new tastes, experimenting with flavor combinations allows you to unlock a world of possibilities and discover your signature vaping experience.

Flavor Pairing Tips:
While there are no hard and fast rules when it comes to mixing flavors in vaping, there are some tips and tricks to help you create balanced and harmonious blends:

Complementary Flavors: Pair flavors that complement each other well to create a cohesive and satisfying vaping experience. For example, pair sweet fruit flavors with creamy dessert flavors or combine tart citrus flavors with refreshing menthol.
Contrast: Experiment with contrasting flavors to create complex and dynamic blends. For example, mix sweet and savory flavors, or combine bold flavors with subtle undertones for a surprising and intriguing vaping experience.
Balance: Achieve balance in your flavor combinations by adjusting the proportions of each flavor to ensure that no single flavor overwhelms the others. Strive for harmony

between the different flavor components to create a well-rounded and enjoyable vaping experience.

Start Small: When experimenting with flavor combinations, start with small batches to test the waters and avoid wasting large quantities of vape juice. This allows you to fine-tune your flavor combinations and make adjustments as needed until you find the perfect blend.

DIY Mixing:

For vapers who enjoy a hands-on approach, DIY mixing offers the ultimate freedom to create custom vape juice blends from scratch. DIY mixing involves combining individual flavor concentrates, PG, VG, and nicotine (if desired) to create unique vape juice recipes tailored to your preferences. With a wide range of flavor concentrates available on the market, DIY mixers can unleash their creativity and craft personalized vape juice blends that are truly one-of-a-kind.

Safety Considerations:

When mixing flavors in vaping, it's essential to prioritize safety and quality. Use high-quality flavor concentrates and ingredients from reputable manufacturers to ensure the safety and purity of your vape juice blends. Follow proper mixing procedures and guidelines to avoid contamination and ensure the integrity of your vape juice. Additionally, be mindful of nicotine levels and handle nicotine-containing ingredients with care to prevent accidental exposure.

In conclusion, mixing and matching flavors in vaping is an exciting and rewarding endeavor that allows vapers to unleash their creativity and customize their vaping experience. Whether you're blending fruity concoctions, decadent desserts, refreshing menthol, or bold tobacco flavors, experimenting with flavor combinations opens up a world of possibilities and allows you to discover new and exciting tastes. With a spirit of experimentation, creativity, and a willingness to explore, vapers can create custom vape juice blends that are as unique and individual as they are.

Customizing Flavors

Customizing Flavors in Vaping

In the world of vaping, customization is key. One of the most exciting aspects of vaping is the ability to tailor the experience to your preferences, and flavor customization plays a significant role in this. Whether you're looking to create a unique flavor combination, replicate a favorite taste, or tweak existing flavors to perfection, the art of customizing flavors opens up a world of possibilities for vapers. Let's explore the process of flavor customization in vaping and how vapers can unleash their creativity to craft personalized vaping experiences:

Flavor Concentrates:
Flavor concentrates are the building blocks of customized vape juice blends. These highly concentrated flavoring agents are available in a wide range of profiles, including fruits, desserts, menthols, tobaccos, and more. Vapers can mix and match flavor concentrates to create unique blends that suit their preferences. With countless flavor options available, the possibilities for flavor customization are virtually endless.

DIY Mixing:
DIY mixing is a popular method of flavor customization among vapers who enjoy a hands-on approach. DIY mixers can purchase individual flavor concentrates, as well as base ingredients such as propylene glycol (PG), vegetable glycerin (VG), and nicotine (if desired), to create custom vape juice blends from scratch. This allows vapers to control every aspect of their vape juice, from flavor intensity to nicotine strength, and tailor it to their exact specifications.

Flavor Enhancement:
Customizing flavors isn't just about creating entirely new blends—it's also about enhancing existing flavors to suit your tastes. Vapers can experiment with adding additional flavor concentrates to pre-made vape juice to intensify or alter the flavor profile. For example, adding a splash of menthol to a fruity blend can create a refreshing twist, while a hint of vanilla can enhance the creaminess of a dessert flavor.

Tailored Nicotine Levels:
Another aspect of flavor customization is adjusting the nicotine level to suit your preferences. Vape juice is available in various nicotine strengths, ranging from nicotine-free to extra high concentrations. By selecting the appropriate nicotine level, vapers can control the intensity of the throat hit and the overall vaping experience. For vapers

looking to reduce their nicotine intake or transition away from nicotine altogether, customizing nicotine levels allows for a gradual and controlled approach.

Flavor Layering:
Flavor layering is a technique used by vapers to create complex and multi-dimensional flavor profiles. By combining multiple flavor concentrates in precise proportions, vapers can achieve a harmonious blend of flavors that evolve with each puff. For example, layering fruity flavors with creamy undertones can create a balanced and nuanced vaping experience that evolves from sweet and tangy to smooth and rich.

Safety and Quality:
When customizing flavors in vaping, it's crucial to prioritize safety and quality. Use high-quality flavor concentrates and ingredients from reputable manufacturers to ensure the purity and integrity of your vape juice blends. Follow proper mixing procedures and guidelines to prevent contamination and ensure the safety of your vape juice. Additionally, be mindful of nicotine handling and storage to prevent accidental exposure.

Flavor Testing and Iteration:
Experimentation is key when customizing flavors in vaping. Don't be afraid to try new combinations and adjust proportions until you find the perfect blend. Keep detailed notes on your recipes and flavor preferences to track your progress and make adjustments as needed. With patience and persistence, you can create custom vape juice blends that are truly one-of-a-kind and perfectly suited to your palate.

In conclusion, flavor customization is an essential aspect of vaping that allows vapers to tailor their vaping experience to their preferences. Whether you're creating entirely new flavor combinations, enhancing existing flavors, or fine-tuning nicotine levels, the art of customizing flavors opens up a world of possibilities for vapers to explore. With creativity, experimentation, and a commitment to quality, vapers can craft personalized vaping experiences that satisfy their taste buds and elevate their enjoyment of vaping.

An Introduction to Vape Coils

Vape coils are an essential component of any vaping device, playing a crucial role in heating the vape juice and producing vapor. Understanding vape coils is essential for vapers who want to optimize their vaping experience and achieve the desired balance of flavor, vapor production, and throat hit. Let's delve into an introduction to vape coils, exploring their construction, function, and different types:

Construction:
Vape coils are typically made from resistance wire, such as Kanthal, stainless steel, nichrome, or nickel, wound into a coil shape. The coil is then encased in a cotton wick, which absorbs vape juice and delivers it to the coil when heated. The coil and wick assembly is housed within the atomizer or coil head, forming the heating element of the vaping device.

Function:
The primary function of a vape coil is to heat the vape juice to the point of vaporization, creating the vapor that is inhaled by the vaper. When the vape device is activated, electricity flows through the coil, generating heat. This heat is transferred to the surrounding cotton wick, causing the vape juice to evaporate and form vapor. The coil's resistance, measured in ohms, determines the amount of heat generated and plays a significant role in the vaping experience.

Types of Vape Coils:
There are several types of vape coils available, each with its unique characteristics and suitability for different vaping styles:

Standard Coils: Standard coils consist of a single wire wrapped into a coil shape, offering a straightforward and reliable heating element. They are commonly used in entry-level vaping devices and provide a balance of flavor and vapor production.
Clapton Coils: Clapton coils are composed of a core wire with a thinner wire wrapped around it in a helical pattern. This design increases the surface area of the coil, resulting in enhanced vapor production and flavor intensity. Clapton coils are popular among cloud chasers and flavor enthusiasts.
Mesh Coils: Mesh coils utilize a mesh-like structure made from resistance wire, offering a larger surface area compared to standard coils. This design allows for faster and more even heating of the vape juice, resulting in improved flavor clarity and vapor production. Mesh coils are known for their smooth and consistent vaping experience.

Ceramic Coils: Ceramic coils feature a ceramic heating element, which provides excellent heat retention and uniform heating of the vape juice. Ceramic coils offer clean and pure flavor, as the ceramic material does not impart any unwanted tastes or odors to the vapor. They are also known for their longevity and durability.

Temperature Control Coils: Temperature control coils are made from specific types of wire, such as stainless steel, nickel, or titanium, that exhibit predictable changes in resistance with temperature. These coils allow vapers to precisely control the temperature of the coil, preventing dry hits and burnt tastes. Temperature control coils are ideal for vapers who prioritize consistency and precision in their vaping experience.

Coil Resistance and Wattage:

Coil resistance, measured in ohms, and wattage play crucial roles in determining the performance of vape coils. Lower resistance coils (sub-ohm coils) require higher wattages to achieve optimal vapor production and flavor intensity, while higher resistance coils require lower wattages. Vapers can adjust the wattage of their device to match the recommended wattage range specified by the coil manufacturer for optimal performance.

Coil Lifespan and Maintenance:

Vape coils have a finite lifespan and will eventually degrade over time due to factors such as heat, oxidation, and buildup of residue from vape juice. Regular maintenance, such as cleaning the coil and changing the cotton wick, can help extend the lifespan of vape coils. Additionally, vapers should be mindful of signs of coil degradation, such as diminished flavor and vapor production, and replace the coil as needed to maintain optimal performance.

In conclusion, vape coils are an essential component of vaping devices that play a crucial role in heating vape juice and producing vapor. Understanding the construction, function, and different types of vape coils is essential for vapers who want to optimize their vaping experience and achieve the desired balance of flavor, vapor production, and throat hit. With a wide range of coil options available, vapers have the flexibility to customize their vaping experience to suit their preferences and vaping style.

Different Types of Coils

Vape coils are the heart of any vaping device, responsible for heating the vape juice and transforming it into the flavorful vapor that vapers enjoy. However, not all coils are created equal, and vapers have a variety of options to choose from when it comes to selecting the right coil for their vaping needs. Understanding the different types of coils available can help vapers make informed decisions and tailor their vaping experience to their preferences. Let's explore some of the most common types of coils used in vaping:

Standard Coils:
Standard coils, also known as single-wire coils, are the simplest and most straightforward type of vape coil. They consist of a single strand of resistance wire, such as Kanthal, wrapped into a coil shape. Standard coils offer reliable performance and are suitable for vapers who prefer a balanced vaping experience with moderate vapor production and flavor intensity. They are commonly used in entry-level vaping devices and provide a hassle-free vaping experience for beginners.

Clapton Coils:
Clapton coils are a popular choice among experienced vapers who are looking to enhance their vaping experience. These coils feature a core wire with a thinner wire wrapped around it in a helical pattern, resembling the structure of a guitar string. Clapton coils offer increased surface area compared to standard coils, resulting in improved vapor production and flavor intensity. The intricate design of Clapton coils allows for faster heating and more efficient vaporization of the vape juice, delivering a smooth and satisfying vaping experience.

Mesh Coils:
Mesh coils have gained popularity in recent years due to their innovative design and superior performance. Instead of using a traditional wire coil, mesh coils utilize a mesh-like structure made from resistance wire, such as Kanthal or stainless steel. Mesh coils offer a larger surface area compared to standard coils, allowing for faster and more even heating of the vape juice. This results in enhanced flavor clarity, smoother vapor production, and reduced ramp-up time. Mesh coils are known for their excellent performance and are favored by cloud chasers and flavor enthusiasts alike.

Ceramic Coils:
Ceramic coils feature a heating element made from porous ceramic material, which provides excellent heat retention and uniform heating of the vape juice. Ceramic coils offer clean and pure flavor, as the ceramic material does not impart any unwanted tastes

or odors to the vapor. Additionally, ceramic coils are known for their longevity and durability, making them a popular choice for vapers who value consistency and reliability in their vaping experience.

Temperature Control Coils:
Temperature control coils are designed specifically for use with temperature control vaping devices, which allow vapers to regulate the temperature of the coil to prevent dry hits and burnt tastes. These coils are typically made from specific types of wire, such as stainless steel, nickel, or titanium, that exhibit predictable changes in resistance with temperature. Temperature control coils offer precise control over the vaping experience and are ideal for vapers who prioritize consistency and accuracy in their vaping experience.

In conclusion, there are several different types of vape coils available, each with its unique characteristics and suitability for different vaping styles. Whether you prefer the simplicity of standard coils, the performance of Clapton or mesh coils, the purity of ceramic coils, or the precision of temperature control coils, there's a vape coil option available to suit your preferences and vaping needs. By understanding the differences between these coil types, vapers can make informed decisions and customize their vaping experience to achieve the perfect balance of flavor, vapor production, and satisfaction.

Learn to Build Your Own Coils

Building your own coils can be an exhilarating and rewarding experience for vapers who are looking to take their vaping journey to the next level. While it may seem daunting at first, learning to build your own coils allows you to customize your vaping experience, fine-tune your device to your preferences, and gain a deeper understanding of the mechanics behind vaping. Here's a comprehensive guide on how to build your own coils:

Gather Your Materials:
Before you begin building your coils, you'll need to gather the necessary materials and tools. These include:

Resistance wire: Choose a wire material such as Kanthal, stainless steel, or nichrome, depending on your preferences.
Coil jig or screwdriver: A coil jig or screwdriver will help you wrap the wire into the desired coil shape.
Wire cutters: Wire cutters are essential for trimming the excess wire and achieving the desired coil length.
Ceramic tweezers: Ceramic tweezers are heat-resistant and allow you to manipulate the coil while it's heating without the risk of short-circuiting.
Ohm reader: An ohm reader is used to measure the resistance of your coils and ensure they are within a safe range for your vaping device.
Choose Your Coil Style:
There are several different coil styles to choose from, each offering its unique characteristics and vaping experience. Some popular coil styles include:

Standard coils: Simple coils consisting of a single wire wrapped into a coil shape.
Clapton coils: Coils with a core wire and a thinner wire wrapped around it in a helical pattern.
Fused Clapton coils: Similar to Clapton coils but with multiple core wires for increased surface area.
Alien coils: Complex coils with a wavy outer wire wrapped around a multi-core wire.
Wrap Your Coils:
Once you've chosen your coil style, it's time to wrap your coils using the resistance wire and coil jig or screwdriver. Start by securing one end of the wire to the jig or screwdriver and wrapping the wire around it in a tight and even manner. The number of wraps will depend on your desired resistance and vaping preferences. Once you've completed the wraps, trim any excess wire with the wire cutters and gently remove the coil from the jig or screwdriver.

Install Your Coils:
After wrapping your coils, it's time to install them into your vaping device's atomizer. Carefully insert the coils into the designated coil posts or slots, ensuring they are positioned evenly and securely. Use the ceramic tweezers to adjust the coils if necessary, ensuring they are aligned and spaced evenly. Once the coils are installed, use the wire cutters to trim any excess wire protruding from the coil posts.

Check Your Resistance:
Before firing your coils, it's essential to check their resistance using an ohm reader. This will ensure that your coils are within a safe range for your vaping device and prevent any potential short circuits or malfunctions. If the resistance is too low or too high, adjust the number of wraps or the gauge of wire used to achieve the desired resistance.

Test and Heat Your Coils:
Once your coils are installed and their resistance is confirmed, it's time to test and heat them. Attach your vaping device to a battery or mod and fire the coils at a low wattage to check for any hotspots or uneven heating. Gently pulse the coils, strumming them with ceramic tweezers to remove any hotspots and ensure they heat evenly from the inside out.

Wick Your Coils:
After heating and testing your coils, it's time to wick them with cotton or another wicking material of your choice. Cut a strip of wicking material and thread it through the center of each coil, ensuring it is snug but not too tight. Trim any excess wick to fit your atomizer's deck and fluff the ends to promote optimal wicking and flavor absorption.

Prime Your Coils and Enjoy:
Before vaping, it's essential to prime your coils by saturating the wicking material with vape juice. Apply a few drops of vape juice to each coil and allow it to soak in for a few minutes. Once the wick is fully saturated, reassemble your atomizer, adjust your airflow and wattage settings, and enjoy your freshly built coils.

Building your own coils may require practice and patience, but the rewards are well worth the effort. Not only does it allow you to customize your vaping experience to your exact preferences, but it also fosters a deeper understanding of the mechanics behind vaping. With the right materials, tools, and techniques, you can become a master coil builder and take your vaping journey to new heights.

Re-wick and Dry Burn Your Coils

Re-wicking and dry burning your coils are essential maintenance tasks that every vaper should master to ensure optimal performance and longevity of their vaping setup. Over time, the wicking material in your coils can become saturated with residue from vape juice, leading to diminished flavor, vapor production, and even unpleasant tastes. Additionally, residue buildup on the coils themselves can cause hotspots and uneven heating, resulting in a less satisfying vaping experience. Re-wicking and dry burning your coils are simple yet effective methods for restoring their performance and extending their lifespan. Here's a comprehensive guide on how to re-wick and dry burn your coils:

Gather Your Materials:
Before you begin re-wicking and dry burning your coils, gather the necessary materials and tools:

Replacement wicking material: Choose a high-quality wicking material such as organic cotton, cotton bacon, or silica wick.
Ceramic tweezers: Ceramic tweezers are heat-resistant and allow you to manipulate the coils while dry burning without the risk of short-circuiting.
Scissors or wire cutters: Scissors or wire cutters are used to trim the wicking material to fit your coils.
Paper towels or a cleaning cloth: Paper towels or a cleaning cloth can be used to wipe down the coils and remove any residue.
Remove the Old Wick:
Start by disassembling your atomizer and removing the old wicking material from the coils. Use the ceramic tweezers to gently pull the wick out of the coil, being careful not to damage the coil itself. Discard the old wick and any residue buildup on the coils.

Clean the Coils:
Once the old wick has been removed, it's time to clean the coils to remove any residue buildup. Dry burning the coils is an effective method for cleaning and rejuvenating them. Attach your atomizer to a battery or mod and fire the coils at a low wattage, pulsing them in short bursts. This will cause any residue on the coils to burn off, leaving them clean and ready for re-wicking.

Trim and Install the New Wick:
After dry burning the coils, trim a strip of replacement wicking material to fit your coils. The wick should be long enough to thread through the center of each coil and reach the bottom of the atomizer's deck. Use the ceramic tweezers to thread the wick through the

coils, ensuring it is snug but not too tight. Trim any excess wick with scissors or wire cutters.

Prime the New Wick:
Before reassembling your atomizer and vaping, it's essential to prime the new wicking material to ensure optimal flavor and vapor production. Apply a few drops of vape juice to each coil, saturating the wick thoroughly. Allow the wick to soak in the vape juice for a few minutes before reassembling your atomizer and adjusting your airflow and wattage settings.

Test and Enjoy:
Once the new wick is primed and your atomizer is reassembled, it's time to test your coils and enjoy your freshly re-wicked setup. Take a few test puffs to ensure that the wicking material is properly saturated and that the coils are heating evenly. Adjust your airflow and wattage settings as needed to achieve your desired vaping experience.

Re-wicking and dry burning your coils are simple yet effective maintenance tasks that can greatly improve the performance and longevity of your vaping setup. By regularly re-wicking your coils and dry burning them to remove residue buildup, you can ensure a clean and satisfying vaping experience every time. With the right materials, tools, and techniques, you can master the art of coil maintenance and enjoy optimal flavor, vapor production, and satisfaction from your vaping device.

Advanced Vaping Techniques

Advanced vaping techniques go beyond the basics of simply inhaling vapor from your device. These techniques involve more intricate methods of manipulating vapor production, flavor intensity, and throat hit to customize your vaping experience according to your preferences. Whether you're a seasoned vaper looking to enhance your vaping journey or a newcomer eager to explore the possibilities, mastering advanced vaping techniques can elevate your enjoyment of vaping to new heights. Let's delve into some of the most popular and effective advanced vaping techniques:

Cloud Chasing:
Cloud chasing is a technique that focuses on maximizing vapor production to create thick, dense clouds of vapor. To achieve impressive clouds, vapers typically use high-powered vaping devices with low-resistance coils and high-VG (vegetable glycerin) vape juice. Increasing airflow by fully opening the device's airflow control and taking long, deep inhales can also enhance cloud production. Advanced cloud chasers may experiment with specialized coil builds, such as Clapton or fused Clapton coils, to further optimize vapor production.

Flavor Boosting:
Flavor boosting techniques aim to intensify the flavor of vape juice, resulting in a more flavorful and enjoyable vaping experience. To enhance flavor, vapers can adjust their vaping device's wattage or temperature settings to find the optimal range for extracting maximum flavor from the vape juice. Using coils with larger surface areas, such as mesh coils, can also enhance flavor by ensuring more even heating of the vape juice. Additionally, experimenting with different vape juice flavors and combinations can help vapers discover new and exciting flavor profiles.

Mouth-to-Lung (MTL) and Direct Lung (DL) Inhales:
Advanced vapers often experiment with different inhaling techniques to achieve varying sensations and experiences. Mouth-to-lung (MTL) inhales involve drawing vapor into the mouth before inhaling it into the lungs, similar to the sensation of smoking a traditional cigarette. MTL inhales are commonly used with higher nicotine concentrations and provide a satisfying throat hit. On the other hand, direct lung (DL) inhales involve inhaling vapor directly into the lungs without holding it in the mouth first. DL inhales are typically used with lower nicotine concentrations and are favored by cloud chasers for their ability to produce large clouds of vapor.

Temperature Control Vaping:

Temperature control vaping is an advanced technique that allows vapers to precisely regulate the temperature of their coils to prevent dry hits and burnt tastes. Temperature control devices monitor the resistance of the coil and adjust power output to maintain a consistent temperature. By setting a specific temperature limit, vapers can prevent the coil from exceeding a certain temperature, resulting in a smoother and more consistent vaping experience. Temperature control vaping is especially beneficial for vapers who use temperature-sensitive coil materials, such as stainless steel, nickel, or titanium.

Coil Building:
Coil building is the process of creating custom coils for your vaping device, allowing for greater control over vapor production, flavor, and throat hit. Advanced vapers often experiment with different coil materials, wire gauges, and coil configurations to achieve their desired vaping experience. Popular coil builds include Clapton coils, fused Clapton coils, alien coils, and staggered coils, each offering unique characteristics and performance benefits. Coil building requires patience, practice, and knowledge of Ohm's law to ensure safe and effective coil designs.

Squonking:
Squonking is a vaping technique that involves using a bottom-feeding (squonk) mod with a specialized atomizer equipped with a built-in juice reservoir. The squonk mod contains a squeezable bottle that allows the vaper to manually pump vape juice into the atomizer's wick and coils as needed. Squonking offers the convenience of a rebuildable dripping atomizer (RDA) with the added benefit of a juice reservoir, eliminating the need to constantly drip vape juice onto the coils.

In conclusion, advanced vaping techniques offer a world of possibilities for vapers to explore and customize their vaping experience according to their preferences. Whether you're interested in chasing clouds, boosting flavor, mastering different inhaling techniques, or experimenting with coil building, there's an advanced vaping technique suited to every vaper's tastes and preferences. With patience, practice, and a willingness to experiment, you can unlock the full potential of your vaping device and enjoy a truly personalized vaping experience.

Sub-Ohm Vaping

Sub-ohm vaping has become increasingly popular among vaping enthusiasts for its ability to produce large clouds of vapor and intense flavor. This advanced vaping technique involves using coils with a resistance of less than one ohm, hence the term "sub-ohm." While sub-ohm vaping offers an exhilarating vaping experience, it's essential to understand its intricacies, benefits, and potential risks.

Enhanced Vapor Production:
Sub-ohm vaping is renowned for its ability to generate massive clouds of vapor. By using coils with lower resistance, sub-ohm vapers can increase the power output of their devices, resulting in faster heating of the coil and more vapor production. This makes sub-ohm vaping an ideal choice for cloud chasers who enjoy performing impressive vape tricks and creating dense plumes of vapor.

Intensified Flavor:
In addition to producing copious amounts of vapor, sub-ohm vaping also enhances the intensity and clarity of flavor. Lower resistance coils allow for more efficient vaporization of the vape juice, resulting in richer and more pronounced flavor profiles. This makes sub-ohm vaping particularly appealing to flavor enthusiasts who appreciate the nuances of different vape juice flavors.

Customizable Experience:
One of the main attractions of sub-ohm vaping is its versatility and customizability. Sub-ohm vapers can fine-tune their vaping experience by adjusting various factors such as coil resistance, wattage, airflow, and vape juice composition. This level of customization allows vapers to tailor their vaping setup to their preferences, whether they prioritize vapor production, flavor intensity, or throat hit.

Potential Risks:
While sub-ohm vaping offers numerous benefits, it's essential to be aware of the potential risks associated with this advanced vaping technique. Sub-ohm vaping requires a significant amount of power, which can put extra strain on the battery and other components of the vaping device. As a result, sub-ohm vapers should use high-quality batteries with a high discharge rate and ensure that their devices are properly maintained to minimize the risk of malfunctions or accidents.

Increased E-Liquid Consumption:

Due to the higher power output and increased vapor production associated with sub-ohm vaping, sub-ohm vapers tend to consume more e-liquid compared to vapers using higher resistance coils. This means that sub-ohm vaping can be more expensive in terms of e-liquid consumption, so vapers should be prepared to replenish their supply of vape juice more frequently.

Importance of Safety Precautions:
Sub-ohm vaping requires a good understanding of Ohm's law and battery safety to ensure a safe and enjoyable vaping experience. It's crucial to use vaping devices and batteries that are compatible with sub-ohm vaping and to follow manufacturer recommendations for coil resistance, wattage, and battery usage. Additionally, vapers should be mindful of proper coil building techniques, proper wicking, and adequate ventilation to prevent overheating and potential hazards.

In conclusion, sub-ohm vaping offers vapers an exciting and customizable vaping experience characterized by enhanced vapor production and intensified flavor. While sub-ohm vaping can be immensely satisfying for those who enjoy chasing clouds and exploring new flavor profiles, it's essential to approach it with caution and prioritize safety. By understanding the principles of sub-ohm vaping, practicing proper safety precautions, and staying informed about the latest advancements in vaping technology, vapers can enjoy the benefits of sub-ohm vaping while minimizing potential risks.

Dripping

Dripping, also known as "dripping atomizers" or "RDA (Rebuildable Dripping Atomizer) vaping," is an advanced vaping technique that has gained popularity among vaping enthusiasts for its ability to deliver intense flavor and vapor production. Unlike traditional tank-style atomizers, which store e-liquid in a reservoir, dripping involves manually dripping e-liquid directly onto the coils and wick of an RDA. While dripping requires a bit more effort than standard vaping methods, many vapers swear by its superior flavor and customizable experience.

Enhanced Flavor:
One of the main attractions of dripping is its ability to deliver unparalleled flavor intensity. By dripping e-liquid directly onto the coils and wick, vapers ensure that the vape juice comes into direct contact with the heating elements, maximizing flavor extraction. This results in a more vibrant and nuanced flavor profile compared to tank-style atomizers, where the e-liquid must travel through a wick and chamber before reaching the coils.

Customizable Experience:
Dripping offers vapers a high degree of customization over their vaping experience. With dripping atomizers, vapers can easily switch between different e-liquid flavors without having to empty and clean a tank. Additionally, dripping allows vapers to adjust factors such as coil resistance, airflow, and wattage to fine-tune their vaping experience according to their preferences. This level of customization appeals to vapers who enjoy experimenting with different vaping setups and optimizing their flavor and vapor production.

Cloud Chasing:
Dripping is particularly popular among cloud chasers, who are vapers that enjoy producing large clouds of vapor. Dripping atomizers are well-suited for cloud chasing due to their ability to handle high-power setups and low-resistance coils. By using specialized coil builds and adjusting airflow settings, vapers can maximize vapor production and perform impressive vape tricks with ease. Dripping is considered the go-to method for cloud chasers who prioritize vapor density and visual appeal in their vaping experience.

Regular Maintenance:
While dripping offers numerous benefits, it also requires regular maintenance to ensure optimal performance. Since dripping atomizers do not have a built-in reservoir for e-

liquid, vapers must manually drip e-liquid onto the coils and wick every few puffs. Additionally, dripping atomizers tend to accumulate residue and gunk from e-liquid and coil buildup more quickly than tank-style atomizers. As a result, vapers should regularly clean and maintain their dripping atomizers to prevent flavor degradation and maintain airflow.

Safety Considerations:
It's essential for vapers to practice proper safety precautions when dripping to minimize the risk of accidents or malfunctions. When building coils for dripping, vapers should ensure that the resistance is within a safe range for their battery and device. Additionally, vapers should be mindful of overheating and avoid chain vaping, which can cause the coils to become too hot and potentially lead to dry hits or burnt tastes. Proper battery safety and maintenance are also crucial to prevent battery failure or venting.

In conclusion, dripping is an advanced vaping technique that offers vapers unparalleled flavor intensity, customization, and cloud production. While dripping requires more effort and maintenance compared to traditional tank-style vaping, many vapers find the superior flavor and vapor production well worth the extra steps. By understanding the principles of dripping and practicing proper safety precautions, vapers can enjoy a highly customizable and satisfying vaping experience with dripping atomizers.

Squonking

Squonking has emerged as a popular vaping trend that combines the convenience of a tank-style atomizer with the flavor and vapor production capabilities of a rebuildable dripping atomizer (RDA). This innovative vaping technique utilizes a special type of vaping device called a squonk mod, paired with a bottom-feeding (squonk) atomizer. Squonking offers vapers the best of both worlds, allowing them to enjoy the benefits of dripping without the hassle of constantly dripping e-liquid onto their coils. Here's everything you need to know about squonking:

How Squonking Works:
At the heart of squonking is the squonk mod, a vaping device equipped with a built-in squeezable bottle (squonk bottle) that contains e-liquid. The squonk mod is typically powered by a single 18650 or 21700 battery and features a specialized 510 connector with a hollow center pin. The squonk atomizer, also known as a bottom-feeding or BF atomizer, is designed with a hollow 510 pin that connects directly to the squonk mod. When the squonk bottle is squeezed, e-liquid is pumped up through the hollow center pin and into the atomizer's deck, saturating the wick and coils with vape juice.

Convenience and Portability:
One of the primary advantages of squonking is its convenience and portability. Unlike traditional dripping atomizers, which require vapers to manually drip e-liquid onto their coils, squonking allows vapers to replenish their vape juice supply with a simple squeeze of the squonk bottle. This eliminates the need to carry around a separate bottle of e-liquid and constantly drip while on the go. Squonk mods are typically compact and ergonomic, making them ideal for vapers who value convenience and portability.

Flavor and Vapor Production:
Squonking offers vapers the same level of flavor intensity and vapor production as traditional dripping atomizers. By delivering e-liquid directly to the coils and wick, squonk atomizers ensure maximum flavor extraction and vaporization. Additionally, squonk mods are compatible with a wide range of coil builds and configurations, allowing vapers to customize their vaping experience to their preferences. Whether you're a flavor enthusiast or a cloud chaser, squonking offers a highly satisfying vaping experience.

Coil Building and Customization:
Squonking opens up a world of possibilities for coil building and customization. Squonk atomizers are compatible with a variety of coil materials, including kanthal, stainless

steel, nickel, and titanium, allowing vapers to experiment with different coil builds and configurations. From simple round wire builds to complex Clapton coils and beyond, squonking offers endless opportunities for vapers to fine-tune their vaping setups and achieve their desired flavor and vapor production.

Safety Considerations:
While squonking offers numerous benefits, it's essential for vapers to prioritize safety when using squonk mods and atomizers. Proper battery safety is crucial to prevent accidents or malfunctions, especially when using mechanical squonk mods. Vapers should ensure that their batteries are properly wrapped, free of any damage, and compatible with their squonk mod's power requirements. Additionally, vapers should be mindful of proper coil building techniques, wicking, and airflow to prevent overheating and potential hazards.

In conclusion, squonking is a highly innovative and convenient vaping technique that offers vapers the best of both worlds. By combining the flavor and vapor production capabilities of dripping atomizers with the convenience of tank-style atomizers, squonking provides vapers with a highly satisfying vaping experience. With its portability, customization options, and flavor intensity, squonking has cemented its place as a popular vaping trend among enthusiasts.

Adjusting Vape Settings for the Best Experience

Adjusting vape settings is a crucial aspect of the vaping experience, allowing users to customize their device to suit their preferences and optimize performance. Whether you're looking to enhance flavor, increase vapor production, or achieve a smoother throat hit, understanding how to adjust vape settings effectively can significantly improve your overall vaping experience. Here's a comprehensive guide on adjusting vape settings for the best experience:

Wattage/Voltage:
One of the most fundamental vape settings to adjust is wattage or voltage. Wattage refers to the amount of power delivered to the coil, while voltage refers to the electrical potential difference between the positive and negative terminals of the battery. Increasing the wattage or voltage can result in higher temperatures and faster coil heating, leading to increased vapor production and potentially stronger flavor. Experimenting with different wattage or voltage settings can help users find their preferred balance between flavor intensity and vapor production.

Temperature Control (TC):
For vapers using temperature control-capable devices and compatible coil materials such as stainless steel, nickel, or titanium, adjusting temperature control settings can provide a more consistent vaping experience. Temperature control allows users to set a specific temperature limit, preventing the coil from exceeding the desired temperature and reducing the risk of dry hits or burnt tastes. By fine-tuning temperature control settings, vapers can enjoy smoother and more flavorful vapor without the risk of overheating the coil.

Airflow:
Adjusting airflow settings can have a significant impact on the vaping experience, affecting both flavor and vapor production. Increasing airflow can result in a cooler vapor and a looser draw, while decreasing airflow can lead to a warmer vapor and a tighter draw. Experimenting with different airflow settings allows users to tailor their vaping experience to their preferences, whether they prefer a more restrictive draw for enhanced flavor or a more open draw for increased vapor production.

Coil Resistance:

Another important vape setting to consider is coil resistance. Coil resistance refers to the amount of resistance the coil presents to the flow of electricity, measured in ohms. Lower resistance coils (sub-ohm coils) generally produce warmer vapor and larger clouds, while higher resistance coils are often favored for mouth-to-lung vaping and enhanced flavor. Adjusting coil resistance can significantly impact the vaping experience, so users should choose coils that match their preferred vaping style and adjust settings accordingly.

Nicotine Strength:
For vapers using nicotine-containing e-liquids, adjusting nicotine strength is essential for achieving the desired level of nicotine satisfaction. Higher nicotine strengths provide a stronger throat hit and faster nicotine delivery, while lower nicotine strengths offer a smoother vaping experience with less throat hit. s should experiment with different nicotine strengths to find the optimal balance between nicotine satisfaction and overall vaping enjoyment.

E-liquid Ratio:
Lastly, adjusting the ratio of vegetable glycerin (VG) to propylene glycol (PG) in e-liquid can also impact the vaping experience. Higher VG ratios typically result in thicker vapor clouds and smoother throat hits, while higher PG ratios offer more intense flavor and a stronger throat hit. s can experiment with different VG/PG ratios to find the ideal balance between vapor production, flavor intensity, and throat hit according to their preferences.

In conclusion, adjusting vape settings is an essential aspect of the vaping experience, allowing users to customize their device to achieve the best possible vaping experience. By experimenting with wattage/voltage, temperature control, airflow, coil resistance, nicotine strength, and e-liquid ratio, vapers can tailor their vaping experience to suit their preferences and enjoy optimal flavor, vapor production, and nicotine satisfaction.

Understanding Wattage, Voltage, and Resistance

Understanding wattage, voltage, and resistance is essential for vapers who want to optimize their vaping experience and achieve their desired flavor, vapor production, and throat hit. These three key factors play a significant role in determining how a vaping device functions and how it delivers vapor to the user. Let's delve deeper into each of these elements:

Wattage:
Wattage refers to the amount of power delivered to the coil in a vaping device. It is measured in watts and determines how quickly the coil heats up and vaporizes the e-liquid. Adjusting the wattage allows vapers to control the temperature of the coil and the intensity of the vaping experience. Higher wattages generally result in hotter coils and more vapor production, while lower wattages produce cooler vapor and less vapor production. Finding the optimal wattage for your vaping device and coil setup is essential for achieving the best balance of flavor and vapor production.

Voltage:
Voltage, like wattage, is a measure of electrical potential difference in a vaping device. It determines the rate at which electrical current flows from the battery to the coil. While wattage takes into account both voltage and resistance, voltage refers specifically to the electrical potential difference between the positive and negative terminals of the battery. Vapers can adjust voltage settings to control the power output of their device and customize their vaping experience. However, it's essential to keep in mind that changing voltage settings without considering coil resistance can lead to inconsistent performance and potential safety hazards.

Resistance:
Resistance is the measure of opposition to the flow of electrical current in a vaping coil. It is measured in ohms and plays a crucial role in determining the wattage and voltage required to achieve a desired vaping experience. Lower resistance coils, also known as sub-ohm coils (coils with a resistance of less than one ohm), generally require higher wattages and voltages to produce vapor, resulting in warmer vapor and larger clouds. Higher resistance coils, on the other hand, require lower wattages and voltages and are often preferred for mouth-to-lung vaping and enhanced flavor.

Understanding the relationship between wattage, voltage, and resistance is essential for vapers to achieve their desired vaping experience safely and effectively. By adjusting these key parameters, vapers can customize their vaping setup to suit their preferences and optimize flavor, vapor production, and throat hit. However, it's crucial to exercise caution when making adjustments to avoid exceeding the limits of your vaping device and battery, which can lead to overheating, coil damage, or other safety hazards.

In conclusion, wattage, voltage, and resistance are fundamental concepts that every vaper should understand to maximize their vaping experience. By mastering these elements and experimenting with different settings, vapers can unlock the full potential of their vaping device and enjoy a highly personalized and satisfying vaping experience. Whether you're a cloud chaser, flavor enthusiast, or throat hit connoisseur, understanding wattage, voltage, and resistance is the key to achieving your vaping goals safely and effectively.

Temperature Control Vaping

Temperature control vaping is an advanced vaping technique that offers vapers greater control over their vaping experience by allowing them to precisely regulate the temperature of their coils. This innovative feature has become increasingly popular among vaping enthusiasts for its ability to provide a more consistent and customized vaping experience while minimizing the risk of dry hits and burnt tastes. Let's explore the ins and outs of temperature control vaping:

How Temperature Control Works:
Temperature control vaping relies on specialized vaping devices equipped with temperature control functionality and compatible coil materials, such as stainless steel, nickel, or titanium. These devices are designed to monitor the temperature of the coil in real-time and automatically adjust power output to maintain a consistent temperature. By setting a specific temperature limit, vapers can prevent the coil from exceeding the desired temperature, resulting in a smoother and more controlled vaping experience.

Benefits of Temperature Control Vaping:
One of the primary benefits of temperature control vaping is its ability to prevent dry hits and burnt tastes. By monitoring and regulating the temperature of the coil, temperature control devices ensure that the e-liquid is vaporized at an optimal temperature, preventing the wick from overheating and drying out. This not only prolongs the life of the coil but also provides vapers with a more consistent and enjoyable vaping experience, free from unpleasant burnt flavors.

Consistency and Customization:
Temperature control vaping offers vapers greater consistency and customization over their vaping experience. Unlike variable wattage vaping, where power output can fluctuate depending on factors such as battery charge and coil resistance, temperature control vaping maintains a steady temperature, resulting in more predictable vapor production and flavor intensity. Additionally, temperature control devices allow vapers to fine-tune their vaping experience by adjusting temperature settings to suit their preferences.

Coil Compatibility and Material:
Temperature control vaping requires the use of compatible coil materials that exhibit predictable changes in resistance with temperature. Stainless steel, nickel, and titanium are commonly used materials for temperature control coils due to their stable resistance characteristics. Vapers should ensure that their coils are made from the appropriate

material and are compatible with their temperature control device to achieve optimal performance.

Safety Considerations:
While temperature control vaping offers numerous benefits, it's essential for vapers to practice proper safety precautions to prevent accidents or malfunctions. Vapers should only use temperature control devices and coils that are specifically designed for temperature control vaping. Additionally, vapers should be mindful of proper coil building techniques, wicking, and airflow to ensure that the coil remains within the desired temperature range and to prevent overheating or potential hazards.

Experimentation and Optimization:
Temperature control vaping provides vapers with the opportunity to experiment with different temperature settings and coil materials to find their preferred vaping experience. By adjusting temperature settings, vapers can fine-tune flavor intensity, vapor production, and throat hit to suit their preferences. Experimenting with different coil materials and temperature ranges allows vapers to unlock new flavor profiles and vaping sensations.

In conclusion, temperature control vaping offers vapers greater control, consistency, and customization over their vaping experience. By regulating the temperature of the coil, temperature control devices provide a smoother and more enjoyable vaping experience while minimizing the risk of dry hits and burnt tastes. Whether you're a flavor enthusiast, cloud chaser, or looking for a more consistent vaping experience, temperature control vaping offers a highly satisfying and customizable option for vapers of all preferences.

Finding Your Ideal Vape Settings

Finding your ideal vape settings is crucial for enjoying a satisfying and personalized vaping experience. With a myriad of options available, including wattage, temperature, airflow, and coil resistance, determining the perfect combination can seem daunting. However, by understanding your preferences and experimenting with different settings, you can discover the setup that best suits your vaping style. Here's how to find your ideal vape settings:

Start with Basic Settings:
If you're new to vaping or trying out a new device, start with the manufacturer's recommended settings. This often includes wattage or voltage ranges suitable for the coil resistance of your atomizer. Following these guidelines can help you get a feel for how your device performs and prevent any potential issues.

Adjust Wattage or Voltage:
Wattage or voltage is a primary setting that determines how much power is delivered to your coil. Experiment with different wattage or voltage levels to find the sweet spot for your preferred flavor and vapor production. Start low and gradually increase the power until you achieve the desired balance of flavor intensity and vapor density.

Explore Temperature Control:
If your device supports temperature control vaping, consider experimenting with this feature. Temperature control allows you to set a specific temperature limit, preventing the coil from overheating and minimizing the risk of dry hits. Start with a moderate temperature and adjust until you find the temperature that provides the best flavor and consistency.

Fine-Tune Airflow:
Airflow plays a crucial role in the vaping experience, affecting both flavor and vapor production. Experiment with different airflow settings to find the level of airflow that suits your preferences. A more restricted airflow can enhance flavor intensity, while a more open airflow can increase vapor production and provide a smoother draw.

Consider Coil Resistance:
Coil resistance, measured in ohms, also influences your vaping experience. Lower resistance coils (sub-ohm coils) generally produce warmer vapor and larger clouds, while higher resistance coils offer a cooler vape with more pronounced flavor. Choose coils that match your preferred vaping style and adjust settings accordingly.

Factor in E-liquid Ratio and Nicotine Strength:
The ratio of vegetable glycerin (VG) to propylene glycol (PG) in your e-liquid, as well as the nicotine strength, can impact your vaping experience. Higher VG ratios produce denser vapor, while higher PG ratios offer more intense flavor and throat hit. Similarly, higher nicotine strengths provide a stronger throat hit and faster nicotine delivery. Experiment with different e-liquid ratios and nicotine strengths to find the combination that best suits your preferences.

Keep Safety in Mind:
While experimenting with vape settings, it's essential to prioritize safety. Avoid exceeding the recommended wattage or temperature limits for your device and coils to prevent overheating and potential hazards. Additionally, ensure that your batteries are properly maintained and compatible with your vaping setup to minimize the risk of accidents.

In conclusion, finding your ideal vape settings is a process of experimentation and discovery. By adjusting wattage, temperature, airflow, coil resistance, e-liquid ratio, and nicotine strength, you can tailor your vaping experience to suit your preferences perfectly. Remember to start with basic settings, explore different options, and prioritize safety throughout your vaping journey. With patience and persistence, you'll find the ideal combination of settings that delivers the ultimate vaping experience for you.

Vaping Etiquette and Culture

Vaping etiquette and culture have evolved alongside the booming popularity of vaping, shaping the way vapers interact with each other and the broader community. As vaping has become more widespread, so too have the norms and practices that govern its social aspects. Understanding vaping etiquette is essential for both seasoned vapers and newcomers to ensure a positive and respectful vaping experience. Let's delve into the world of vaping etiquette and culture:

Respect Others' Space:
One of the cardinal rules of vaping etiquette is to be mindful of others' personal space and comfort. While many people enjoy the aroma of flavored vapor, not everyone may share the same sentiment. Be considerate when vaping in public spaces, such as restaurants, public transportation, or crowded areas. Always ask for permission before vaping in someone else's space, and be willing to accommodate their preferences.

Follow Applicable Laws and Regulations:
Vaping regulations vary from one region to another, with some areas imposing restrictions on where and when vaping is permitted. It's crucial to familiarize yourself with local vaping laws and regulations to avoid inadvertently violating them. Respect designated vaping areas and adhere to any signage indicating where vaping is allowed or prohibited.

Practice Common Courtesy:
Just as with smoking, common courtesy dictates that vapers should refrain from vaping in enclosed spaces where others may be exposed to secondhand vapor. Additionally, avoid vaping in situations where it may be disruptive or distracting to others, such as during meetings, lectures, or social gatherings where vaping is not the focal point.

Dispose of Waste Responsibly:
Proper disposal of vape-related waste, such as empty e-liquid bottles, used coils, and packaging, is an integral part of vaping etiquette. Dispose of waste responsibly in designated receptacles or recycling bins to help maintain a clean and tidy environment. Avoid littering or leaving vape-related waste in public spaces, as it reflects poorly on the vaping community as a whole.

Be Inclusive and Welcoming:
Vaping culture is built on a sense of community and camaraderie among vapers. Embrace inclusivity and be welcoming to vapers of all backgrounds, experiences, and preferences.

Share knowledge, offer support, and engage in constructive discussions with fellow vapers to foster a positive and supportive vaping community.

Practice Battery Safety:
Battery safety is paramount in vaping culture to prevent accidents or malfunctions. Always use high-quality batteries from reputable manufacturers and avoid using damaged or expired batteries. Familiarize yourself with battery safety best practices, such as proper storage, handling, and charging, to minimize the risk of battery-related incidents.

Educate Others Responsibly:
As a vaper, you may encounter individuals who are curious about vaping or have misconceptions about it. Take the opportunity to educate others responsibly by sharing accurate information and dispelling myths about vaping. However, be mindful not to pressure or influence others to vape if they are not interested or comfortable doing so.

In conclusion, vaping etiquette and culture encompass a range of practices and norms that contribute to a positive and respectful vaping experience for all. By adhering to principles of respect, courtesy, responsibility, and inclusivity, vapers can help cultivate a thriving and supportive vaping community. Whether you're a seasoned vaper or new to the vaping scene, embracing vaping etiquette is essential for fostering a culture of mutual respect and understanding within the vaping community.

Do's and Don'ts of Vaping

Vaping has become increasingly popular in recent years, with millions of people worldwide embracing it as an alternative to traditional smoking. While vaping offers numerous benefits, it's essential to understand the do's and don'ts to ensure a safe, enjoyable, and responsible vaping experience. Whether you're new to vaping or a seasoned enthusiast, here are some important guidelines to keep in mind:

Do's:

Do Familiarize Yourself with Your Vaping Device:
Before using your vaping device, take the time to read the user manual thoroughly and familiarize yourself with its features, functions, and safety precautions. Understanding how your device works will help you use it more effectively and prevent accidents or malfunctions.

Do Practice Battery Safety:
Battery safety is paramount in vaping. Always use high-quality batteries from reputable manufacturers and avoid using damaged or expired batteries. Properly store, handle, and charge your batteries to minimize the risk of battery-related incidents.

Do Experiment with Different E-liquids and Flavors:
One of the joys of vaping is the vast array of e-liquid flavors available. Experiment with different flavors and e-liquid ratios to discover your favorites. Keep an open mind and explore new flavors to enhance your vaping experience.

Do Stay Hydrated:
Vaping can sometimes cause mild dehydration due to the ingredients in e-liquids. Stay hydrated by drinking plenty of water, especially if you find yourself vaping frequently throughout the day. Keeping hydrated will help maintain your overall well-being and prevent dehydration-related issues.

Do Practice Proper Vaping Etiquette:
Be considerate of others when vaping in public spaces. Always ask for permission before vaping in someone else's space, and be mindful of designated vaping areas and any applicable laws or regulations. Dispose of vape-related waste responsibly to maintain a clean and tidy environment.

Don'ts:

Don't Vape in Restricted Areas:
Respect designated vaping areas and adhere to any signage indicating where vaping is allowed or prohibited. Avoid vaping in enclosed spaces where others may be exposed to secondhand vapor, such as restaurants, public transportation, or crowded areas.

Don't Ignore Battery Warnings:
Pay attention to any warning signs or indicators from your vaping device, such as low battery warnings or error messages. Ignoring these warnings can lead to potential safety hazards or damage to your device. Replace or recharge batteries as needed and address any issues promptly.

Don't Overlook Coil Maintenance:
Regularly inspect and clean your coils to ensure optimal performance and flavor. Avoid using coils that are worn out, damaged, or covered in residue, as they can affect the quality of your vaping experience. Replace coils as needed to maintain flavor and vapor production.

Don't Exceed Recommended Wattage or Temperature Limits:
Stay within the recommended wattage or temperature limits for your device and coils to prevent overheating and potential hazards. Exceeding these limits can lead to burnt tastes, coil damage, or even battery failure. Follow manufacturer guidelines and exercise caution when adjusting settings.

Don't Vape if You're Underage or Non-smoking:
Vaping is intended for adults of legal smoking age and should not be used by underage individuals or non-smokers. If you're underage or have never smoked before, refrain from vaping to avoid potential health risks and nicotine dependence.

In conclusion, following these do's and don'ts of vaping will help you enjoy a safe, responsible, and enjoyable vaping experience. By prioritizing safety, respecting others, and practicing good vaping etiquette, you can contribute to a positive vaping culture and community. Whether you're a novice vaper or an experienced enthusiast, incorporating these guidelines into your vaping routine will help ensure a fulfilling and satisfying vaping experience.

Understanding Vape Culture

Vape culture has emerged as a vibrant and diverse community of individuals who share a passion for vaping and the culture surrounding it. This culture encompasses a wide range of attitudes, behaviors, and rituals that have developed around the practice of vaping. Understanding vape culture is essential for both newcomers and seasoned vapers alike, as it offers insight into the social, recreational, and even artistic aspects of vaping. Here's a closer look at what vape culture entails:

Social Connection:
Vape culture is deeply rooted in social connections and camaraderie among vapers. Vaping enthusiasts often gather at vape shops, conventions, and online forums to share experiences, swap tips, and discuss their favorite devices and e-liquids. These social interactions foster a sense of community and belonging among vapers, regardless of their backgrounds or preferences.

Creativity and Innovation:
Vape culture embraces creativity and innovation, with vapers constantly experimenting with new devices, e-liquid flavors, and coil builds. From customizing vape mods to creating intricate coil designs, vapers showcase their creativity through their vaping setups and accessories. The ever-evolving nature of vape culture drives manufacturers to push the boundaries of design and technology, resulting in a diverse array of vaping products and innovations.

Artistic Expression:
Vape culture intersects with art in various forms, from vape trick competitions to vape-related artwork and photography. Vapers showcase their skills and creativity through intricate vape tricks, such as blowing O's, jellyfish, and tornadoes. Vape photography has also gained popularity on social media platforms, with vapers capturing visually stunning images of their vaping setups and clouds.

Advocacy and Education:
Vape culture encompasses a strong advocacy and education component, with vapers advocating for their rights to access harm reduction alternatives to smoking. Vape enthusiasts often engage in grassroots advocacy efforts, such as contacting legislators, attending rallies, and raising awareness about the benefits of vaping as a smoking cessation tool. Education is also a key aspect of vape culture, with vapers sharing evidence-based information about vaping safety, regulations, and best practices.

Diversity and Inclusivity:
Vape culture celebrates diversity and inclusivity, welcoming vapers of all backgrounds, experiences, and preferences. Whether you're a cloud chaser, flavor enthusiast, or mouth-to-lung vaper, there's a place for you in the vape community. Vape culture embraces diversity in vaping styles, e-liquid preferences, and vaping setups, fostering an inclusive environment where everyone can find their niche.

Rituals and Traditions:
Vape culture has its own set of rituals and traditions that vapers engage in as part of their vaping experience. From coil building and wicking to cloud competitions and vape meets, these rituals add depth and meaning to the vaping community. Vapers often develop personal rituals around their vaping routine, such as sampling new e-liquids, cleaning their devices, or attending vape events.

In conclusion, vape culture is a multifaceted and dynamic community that encompasses social connections, creativity, advocacy, and diversity. Understanding vape culture provides insight into the shared values, traditions, and experiences that unite vapers around the world. Whether you're drawn to vaping for its social aspect, artistic expression, or harm reduction potential, vape culture offers a welcoming and inclusive space where enthusiasts can connect, learn, and celebrate their shared passion for vaping.

Participating in Vape Communities

Participating in vape communities is a fantastic way for vaping enthusiasts to connect, share experiences, and stay informed about the latest trends and developments in the world of vaping. Whether you're a beginner looking for guidance or an experienced vaper eager to share your knowledge, vape communities offer a supportive and inclusive environment for vapers of all levels. Here's a closer look at how you can get involved in vape communities and make the most of your vaping journey:

Online Forums and Social Media Groups:
Online forums and social media groups dedicated to vaping are bustling hubs of activity where vapers gather to discuss everything from device recommendations to e-liquid flavors and coil building techniques. Platforms like Reddit, E-Cigarette Forum (ECF), and Facebook groups provide spaces for vapers to ask questions, share tips, and connect with like-minded individuals from around the world. Joining these communities allows you to tap into a wealth of knowledge and expertise while forming valuable connections with fellow vapers.

Vape Meetups and Events:
Vape meetups and events are excellent opportunities to meet fellow vapers in person, exchange vaping stories, and try out new products. These gatherings often feature cloud competitions, giveaways, and vendor booths showcasing the latest vaping gear and accessories. Keep an eye out for local vape meetups or larger-scale vaping conventions in your area, and don't hesitate to attend and immerse yourself in the vibrant vape community.

Vape Shops and Lounges:
Vape shops and lounges serve as community hubs where vapers can not only purchase vaping supplies but also engage with knowledgeable staff and fellow customers. Many vape shops host vape nights, tasting events, or build workshops where vapers can come together to learn, socialize, and bond over their shared passion for vaping. Visiting your local vape shop regularly can help you build relationships with other vapers and stay connected to the local vape scene.

Online Reviewers and Influencers:
Following online reviewers and influencers in the vaping community is another way to stay informed and engaged. These individuals often share comprehensive reviews, tutorials, and vaping-related content on platforms like YouTube, Instagram, and blogs. By subscribing to their channels or following their profiles, you can stay up-to-date on

the latest vaping products, trends, and industry news while learning valuable tips and tricks from seasoned vapers.

Advocacy and Support Groups:
Vaping advocacy and support groups play a vital role in fighting for vapers' rights and promoting harm reduction alternatives to smoking. Organizations like the Consumer Advocates for Smoke-Free Alternatives Association (CASAA) and the Vaping Advocacy and Education Project (VAEP) advocate for sensible vaping regulations and provide resources for vapers looking to get involved in advocacy efforts. Joining these groups allows you to contribute to the broader vaping community while advocating for policies that support vaping access and awareness.

In conclusion, participating in vape communities offers numerous benefits, from gaining knowledge and support to forming meaningful connections with fellow vapers. Whether you're engaging in online forums, attending vape meetups, or supporting advocacy efforts, being an active member of the vape community enriches your vaping experience and strengthens the community as a whole. So don't hesitate to dive in, connect with fellow vapers, and immerse yourself in the vibrant world of vaping communities.

Troubleshooting Common Vape Issues

Troubleshooting common vape issues is an essential skill for every vaper to master. From minor annoyances like leaking tanks to more serious concerns like burnt coils, understanding how to diagnose and fix these problems can save you time, money, and frustration. Here's a comprehensive guide to troubleshooting some of the most common vape issues:

Leaking Tanks:
Leaking tanks are a common issue that can result from several factors, including improper assembly, worn-out seals, or overfilling. To troubleshoot a leaking tank, disassemble it and check for any visible signs of damage or wear on the O-rings and seals. Ensure that all components are properly tightened and seated, and avoid overfilling the tank to prevent excess pressure buildup.

Burnt or Dry Hits:
Burnt or dry hits occur when the coil heats up without enough e-liquid to vaporize, resulting in a harsh, unpleasant taste. This can be caused by insufficient wicking, a depleted e-liquid supply, or high wattage settings. To address this issue, check the wicking material to ensure it is properly saturated with e-liquid. Lowering the wattage or using a higher resistance coil can also help prevent dry hits.

Gurgling or Flooding:
Gurgling or flooding occurs when excess e-liquid accumulates in the coil and airflow chamber, leading to a gurgling sound or spitting of e-liquid into the mouth. This can be caused by overfilling the tank, improper coil installation, or a flooded coil. To resolve this issue, disassemble the tank and remove any excess e-liquid. Check the coil and ensure it is properly seated and not flooded with e-liquid.

Weak Flavor or Vapor Production:
Weak flavor or vapor production can be attributed to various factors, including worn-out coils, improper airflow settings, or expired e-liquid. To troubleshoot this issue, replace the coil if it is old or worn out and adjust the airflow to optimize flavor and vapor production. Additionally, ensure that your e-liquid is fresh and stored properly to maintain its quality and flavor.

Battery Issues:
Battery issues, such as short battery life or inconsistent performance, can affect your vaping experience. This may be caused by a depleted battery, improper charging habits,

or a faulty battery connection. To address battery issues, charge your batteries fully before use and avoid overcharging or discharging them completely. Clean the battery contacts regularly to ensure a secure connection with the device.

No Vapor Production:
If your device is not producing any vapor, check for common issues such as a depleted e-liquid supply, a faulty coil, or a loose connection. Ensure that the tank is properly filled with e-liquid and that the coil is installed correctly. Check the device for any signs of damage or malfunction and troubleshoot accordingly.

Strange Tastes or Smells:
Strange tastes or smells can indicate contamination of the e-liquid or coil, improper coil installation, or coil degradation. To address this issue, clean the tank thoroughly and replace the coil if necessary. Ensure that your e-liquid is fresh and stored properly to prevent contamination and maintain flavor integrity.

In conclusion, troubleshooting common vape issues is an essential skill for vapers of all levels. By understanding the underlying causes of these issues and implementing effective troubleshooting techniques, you can resolve problems quickly and enjoy a smooth and satisfying vaping experience. If you encounter persistent or serious issues, don't hesitate to seek assistance from knowledgeable vapers or vape shop professionals for further guidance and support.

Leaking Tank and Burnt Coils

Dealing with a leaking tank and burnt coils is a common frustration among vapers, but understanding the causes and solutions for these issues can significantly improve your vaping experience. Leaking tanks and burnt coils can disrupt your enjoyment of vaping, leading to wasted e-liquid, unpleasant tastes, and overall dissatisfaction. However, with some troubleshooting and preventive measures, you can minimize these problems and enjoy a smoother vaping experience.

Leaking Tank:

Leaking tanks are a widespread issue in the vaping community, but they can be addressed with some simple steps. One of the most common causes of a leaking tank is improper assembly or a faulty seal. If your tank is leaking, the first step is to disassemble it and inspect the O-rings and seals for any signs of damage or wear. Replace any damaged seals to ensure a proper seal between the tank components.

Another common cause of leaking tanks is overfilling. When you overfill your tank, it creates excess pressure that can force e-liquid to leak out through the airflow holes. To prevent overfilling, follow the manufacturer's guidelines for filling your tank and avoid exceeding the maximum fill linc.

Additionally, changes in temperature or air pressure can sometimes cause a tank to leak. If you notice that your tank is leaking more in certain conditions, such as hot weather or after flying on an airplane, try storing your device upright and avoiding extreme temperature changes.

Burnt Coils:

Burnt coils are another frustrating issue that can occur with vaping, but they are often preventable with proper maintenance and care. A burnt taste when vaping is usually a sign that your coil has reached the end of its lifespan or has been damaged in some way.

One common cause of burnt coils is vaping at too high a wattage. When you exceed the recommended wattage for your coil, it can cause the wicking material to burn, resulting in a burnt taste. To prevent this, always start at a lower wattage and gradually increase until you find the optimal setting for your coil.

Another cause of burnt coils is chain vaping, which can lead to the wicking material becoming dry and burnt. Give your coil time to re-saturate with e-liquid between puffs to prevent this from happening.

Using e-liquids with high levels of sweetener can also contribute to burnt coils, as the sweetener can caramelize and build up on the coil over time. Opt for e-liquids with lower sweetener content to prolong the life of your coils.

Regularly cleaning and maintaining your tank can also help prevent burnt coils. Clean your tank and replace your coils regularly to ensure optimal performance and flavor.

In conclusion, dealing with a leaking tank and burnt coils can be frustrating, but understanding the causes and taking preventive measures can help minimize these issues. By properly assembling your tank, avoiding overfilling, vaping at the correct wattage, and using high-quality e-liquids, you can enjoy a smoother and more satisfying vaping experience with fewer problems.

Battery Issues

Battery issues are a common concern for vapers that can disrupt their vaping experience and pose safety risks if not addressed properly. Understanding the potential causes of battery issues and how to troubleshoot them is crucial for ensuring safe and enjoyable vaping sessions.

One of the most common battery issues encountered by vapers is short battery life. Several factors can contribute to this problem, including the age and quality of the battery, the wattage settings used, and the frequency of vaping. Over time, rechargeable batteries lose their capacity to hold a charge, resulting in shorter battery life. Additionally, vaping at higher wattages or using sub-ohm coils can drain the battery more quickly. To address short battery life, vapers should invest in high-quality batteries from reputable manufacturers and consider carrying spare batteries or a portable charging device for extended vaping sessions.

Another common battery issue is inconsistent performance, which may manifest as uneven power output, sudden drops in battery level, or failure to hold a charge. Inconsistent performance can be caused by various factors, including poor battery maintenance, overcharging, or a faulty connection between the battery and the vaping device. To troubleshoot this issue, vapers should check the battery contacts for dirt or debris and clean them regularly to ensure a secure connection. Additionally, avoiding overcharging or discharging the battery completely can help prolong its lifespan and maintain consistent performance.

Safety is paramount when it comes to vaping batteries, as mishandling or neglecting battery care can result in potentially dangerous situations such as overheating, venting, or even explosions. One of the most important safety precautions for vapers is to use batteries that are specifically designed for vaping and have the appropriate specifications for their device. Using incompatible or damaged batteries can pose serious safety risks and should be avoided at all costs.

Proper battery care and maintenance are essential for preventing battery issues and ensuring safe vaping practices. Vapers should store their batteries in a cool, dry place away from direct sunlight and extreme temperatures to prevent degradation. It is also crucial to avoid exposing batteries to water or other liquids, as this can damage the battery and pose safety risks.

Additionally, vapers should always use the correct charger for their batteries and avoid leaving them unattended while charging. Overcharging can lead to overheating and damage the battery, so it is essential to monitor the charging process and remove the battery from the charger once fully charged.

In conclusion, understanding battery issues and how to address them is essential for vapers to enjoy a safe and satisfying vaping experience. By investing in high-quality batteries, practicing proper battery care and maintenance, and following safety precautions, vapers can minimize the risk of battery issues and enjoy worry-free vaping sessions.

Vape Device Not Producing Vapor

Experiencing a vape device that's not producing vapor can be frustrating, especially when you're craving that satisfying cloud. However, understanding the potential causes behind this issue can help you troubleshoot and get back to enjoying your vaping experience.

One common reason for a vape device not producing vapor is an empty or low e-liquid level. If your tank is running low on e-liquid, there may not be enough liquid to vaporize, resulting in little to no vapor production. To address this, simply refill your tank with fresh e-liquid and ensure that it's adequately saturated with the coil's wicking material.

Another possible cause is a faulty or worn-out coil. Over time, coils can degrade and lose their ability to vaporize e-liquid effectively, resulting in poor vapor production. If you suspect that your coil may be the culprit, try replacing it with a new one. Be sure to prime the new coil properly by saturating the wicking material with e-liquid before use to prevent dry hits and extend its lifespan.

Additionally, insufficient airflow can hinder vapor production by restricting the flow of air through the device. Check your device's airflow settings to ensure that they're open and unrestricted. Adjusting the airflow to a more open setting can help increase vapor production by allowing for better airflow through the coil and tank.

Another factor to consider is the wattage or power settings on your device. Vaping at too low a wattage may not provide enough power to vaporize the e-liquid efficiently, resulting in weak vapor production. Conversely, vaping at too high a wattage can lead to burnt or dry hits. Experiment with adjusting the wattage settings on your device to find the optimal range for your preferred vaping experience.

It's also essential to ensure that your battery is adequately charged, as a low battery level can affect the device's ability to produce vapor. If your battery is running low, recharge it using the appropriate charger for your device. Additionally, check for any loose connections between the battery and the device, as poor connections can interfere with power delivery and affect vapor production.

Finally, cleanliness is key when it comes to maintaining optimal vapor production. A dirty or gunked-up coil can impede vapor production by inhibiting the flow of e-liquid to the heating element. Regularly clean your device and replace coils as needed to ensure peak performance and vapor production.

In conclusion, a vape device not producing vapor can be caused by a variety of factors, including low e-liquid levels, faulty coils, restricted airflow, improper wattage settings, low battery levels, and dirty components. By troubleshooting these potential issues and addressing them accordingly, you can quickly resolve the issue and get back to enjoying your vaping experience. Remember to practice proper maintenance and care for your device to ensure consistent and satisfying vapor production over time.

Health Concerns and Vaping

Health concerns surrounding vaping have been a topic of debate and discussion since the advent of e-cigarettes. While vaping is often touted as a safer alternative to traditional smoking, there are still valid concerns about its potential health impacts. Understanding these concerns and the current state of research can help vapers make informed decisions about their vaping habits.

One of the primary health concerns associated with vaping is the inhalation of potentially harmful chemicals and toxins present in e-cigarette aerosols. While e-cigarettes do not contain tobacco or produce tar like traditional cigarettes, they do contain other chemicals such as nicotine, propylene glycol, glycerin, and flavorings. Some of these chemicals have been linked to respiratory issues, cardiovascular problems, and other health risks when inhaled in high concentrations or over a prolonged period.

Nicotine addiction is another significant health concern associated with vaping. Nicotine is a highly addictive substance that can lead to dependence and withdrawal symptoms when not consumed regularly. While some vapers use e-cigarettes as a tool to quit smoking or reduce their nicotine intake, others may inadvertently become addicted to nicotine through vaping.

Additionally, there have been reports of serious lung injuries and respiratory illnesses associated with vaping, particularly among users of illicit or counterfeit vaping products. These cases, often referred to as vaping-related lung injuries (EVALI), have raised alarms about the safety of vaping and underscore the importance of purchasing vaping products from reputable sources and avoiding black market or counterfeit products.

Furthermore, there is ongoing debate and research surrounding the long-term health effects of vaping. While some studies suggest that vaping may be less harmful than smoking traditional cigarettes and could potentially help smokers quit, others raise concerns about the potential risks of inhaling e-cigarette aerosols and the unknown effects of long-term vaping use.

It's essential for vapers to be aware of these health concerns and take steps to mitigate potential risks. Here are some tips for reducing health risks associated with vaping:

Choose reputable brands and products: Purchase vaping products from trusted manufacturers and retailers to ensure product quality and safety.

Avoid black market or counterfeit products: Stick to regulated vaping products and avoid purchasing vaping products from unlicensed or unauthorized sellers.

Monitor nicotine intake: Be mindful of your nicotine consumption and consider gradually reducing nicotine levels if you're trying to quit smoking or reduce dependence.

Practice proper vaping techniques: Follow manufacturer guidelines for device use and maintenance, and avoid modifying or tampering with vaping devices.

Stay informed: Stay up-to-date on the latest research and developments in vaping and make informed decisions about your vaping habits based on scientific evidence and expert recommendations.

In conclusion, while vaping may offer certain advantages over traditional smoking, there are valid health concerns associated with vaping that should not be overlooked. By understanding these concerns and taking proactive steps to mitigate potential risks, vapers can make informed choices about their vaping habits and prioritize their health and well-being.

Risks and Benefits of Vaping

The practice of vaping, or using electronic cigarettes to inhale aerosolized liquids, has become increasingly popular in recent years as an alternative to traditional smoking. As with any activity involving the inhalation of substances into the lungs, there are both risks and potential benefits associated with vaping. Understanding these factors is crucial for individuals considering vaping as well as those already engaged in the practice.

Risks:

Health Concerns: One of the primary risks associated with vaping is the potential health effects of inhaling aerosolized chemicals and toxins. While e-cigarettes do not produce tar like traditional cigarettes, they do contain other harmful substances such as nicotine, propylene glycol, glycerin, and flavorings. Long-term inhalation of these substances may lead to respiratory issues, cardiovascular problems, and other health risks.

Nicotine Addiction: Nicotine, a highly addictive substance found in many vaping products, poses a significant risk of addiction for users. Regular vaping can lead to nicotine dependence, making it challenging to quit or reduce vaping habits. Nicotine addiction can have detrimental effects on physical and mental health, as well as financial implications due to ongoing expenses associated with vaping.

Potential for Lung Injuries: In recent years, there have been reports of serious lung injuries and respiratory illnesses linked to vaping, particularly among users of illicit or counterfeit vaping products. These cases, often referred to as vaping-related lung injuries (EVALI), have raised concerns about the safety of vaping and underscore the importance of using regulated and reputable vaping products.

Benefits:

Smoking Cessation Aid: One of the most commonly cited benefits of vaping is its potential as a smoking cessation aid. Many smokers turn to vaping as a less harmful alternative to traditional smoking, with some using e-cigarettes to gradually reduce their nicotine intake and eventually quit smoking altogether. While more research is needed to fully understand the effectiveness of vaping as a smoking cessation tool, some studies suggest that it may be helpful for certain individuals looking to quit smoking.

Reduced Harm: Compared to traditional cigarettes, e-cigarettes are generally considered to be less harmful due to the absence of tobacco and tar. Vaping eliminates the combustion process associated with smoking, which produces harmful chemicals and carcinogens. While vaping still carries some health risks, it may be a safer option for individuals who are unable or unwilling to quit smoking using other methods.

Flavors and Customization: Vaping offers a wide variety of flavors and customization options, allowing users to tailor their vaping experience to their preferences. From fruity and dessert-inspired flavors to different nicotine strengths and device types, vapers have the flexibility to experiment and find what works best for them. This customization aspect of vaping can enhance enjoyment and satisfaction for many users.

In conclusion, vaping presents both risks and potential benefits, and individuals should carefully weigh these factors when considering whether to engage in the practice. While vaping may offer certain advantages such as harm reduction and smoking cessation support, it also carries risks such as nicotine addiction and potential health effects. By staying informed and making informed choices, individuals can maximize the potential benefits of vaping while minimizing associated risks.

Vaping and Smoking: A Comparison

Vaping and smoking are two popular methods of consuming nicotine, but they differ significantly in their delivery mechanisms, health effects, and overall user experience. Understanding the differences between vaping and smoking is essential for individuals looking to make informed decisions about their nicotine consumption habits.

Delivery Mechanism:

Vaping involves inhaling aerosolized vapor produced by heating e-liquid (also known as vape juice) in an electronic cigarette or vape device. The e-liquid typically contains nicotine, flavorings, and other additives suspended in a base of propylene glycol and vegetable glycerin. When heated, the e-liquid vaporizes and is inhaled by the user, delivering nicotine to the bloodstream through the lungs.

Smoking, on the other hand, involves burning tobacco and inhaling the resulting smoke into the lungs. The smoke contains thousands of harmful chemicals and carcinogens, including tar, carbon monoxide, and ammonia. These chemicals are produced by the combustion process and can have detrimental effects on respiratory health and overall well-being.

Health Effects:

One of the most significant differences between vaping and smoking is their respective health effects. Smoking is widely recognized as a leading cause of preventable death and disease worldwide, responsible for a range of serious health conditions such as lung cancer, heart disease, and respiratory illnesses. The harmful chemicals and carcinogens present in cigarette smoke contribute to the development of these conditions, making smoking a major public health concern.

In contrast, vaping is generally considered to be less harmful than smoking due to the absence of combustion and tobacco. While e-cigarettes still contain nicotine and other potentially harmful substances, they produce fewer harmful chemicals and carcinogens compared to traditional cigarettes. Research suggests that switching from smoking to vaping may lead to improvements in respiratory function and overall health for some individuals, although more long-term studies are needed to fully understand the health effects of vaping.

Experience:

The user experience of vaping and smoking also differs significantly. Vaping offers a wide variety of flavors and customization options, allowing users to tailor their vaping experience to their preferences. From fruity and dessert-inspired flavors to different nicotine strengths and device types, vapers have the flexibility to experiment and find what works best for them. Additionally, vaping eliminates many of the social and environmental drawbacks associated with smoking, such as lingering odor, ash, and secondhand smoke.

Smoking, on the other hand, is often associated with a strong odor, yellowing of teeth and fingers, and social stigma. Many smokers report feeling ostracized or judged by non-smokers due to the negative health effects and societal attitudes towards smoking. Additionally, smoking restrictions and bans in public places further limit where smokers can indulge in their habit, leading to inconvenience and frustration for many.

In conclusion, while vaping and smoking both involve the consumption of nicotine, they differ significantly in their delivery mechanisms, health effects, and user experience. Vaping is generally considered to be less harmful than smoking and offers greater customization and flexibility for users. However, both vaping and smoking carry risks, and individuals should carefully consider these factors when choosing how to consume nicotine.

Addressing Vaping Myths

Addressing Vaping Myths

As vaping continues to gain popularity as an alternative to traditional smoking, it has also become the subject of numerous myths and misconceptions. While some of these myths may be rooted in misunderstandings or misinformation, others are perpetuated by sensationalized media coverage and anti-vaping advocacy groups. In this article, we'll debunk some of the most common vaping myths and provide evidence-based information to help separate fact from fiction.

Myth 1: Vaping is just as harmful as smoking.

Fact: While vaping is not entirely risk-free, research suggests that it is significantly less harmful than smoking traditional cigarettes. Unlike smoking, which involves the combustion of tobacco and the inhalation of thousands of harmful chemicals and carcinogens, vaping does not produce tar or other harmful byproducts of combustion. While e-cigarette aerosols may contain some potentially harmful substances such as nicotine and flavorings, they are generally considered to be less harmful than cigarette smoke. Numerous studies have shown that smokers who switch to vaping experience improvements in respiratory function and overall health.

Myth 2: Vaping is a gateway to smoking for young people.

Fact: There is limited evidence to support the notion that vaping serves as a gateway to smoking for young people. While it is true that some young people who vape may later try smoking, the vast majority of youth who experiment with vaping do not go on to become regular smokers. In fact, studies have shown that vaping rates among young people have been declining in recent years, even as smoking rates continue to decline. Additionally, many young people who vape do so as a means of avoiding or quitting smoking traditional cigarettes.

Myth 3: Secondhand vapor is just as harmful as secondhand smoke.

Fact: Secondhand vapor from e-cigarettes contains significantly lower levels of harmful chemicals and carcinogens compared to secondhand smoke from traditional cigarettes. While e-cigarette aerosols may contain some potentially harmful substances such as nicotine and ultrafine particles, they are present at much lower levels than those found in cigarette smoke. Numerous studies have shown that exposure to secondhand vapor poses minimal risk to bystanders, especially in well-ventilated indoor spaces.

Myth 4: Vaping is just as addictive as smoking.

Fact: While vaping products contain nicotine, which is an addictive substance, they do not deliver nicotine in the same way as traditional cigarettes. Unlike smoking, which involves the rapid delivery of nicotine to the bloodstream through the lungs, vaping delivers nicotine more slowly and at lower concentrations. As a result, vaping is generally considered to be less addictive than smoking, and many vapers report that they are able to reduce or quit vaping more easily than smoking.

Myth 5: Vaping is only for smokers trying to quit.

Fact: While many people use vaping as a smoking cessation aid, it is also used by non-smokers and former smokers for other reasons, such as nicotine replacement therapy, harm reduction, or simply as a recreational activity. Some non-smokers use vaping as a way to experiment with different flavors or to socialize with friends who vape. Additionally, many former smokers continue to vape long after quitting smoking as a way to satisfy their nicotine cravings without the harmful effects of smoking.

In conclusion, vaping myths abound, but many of them are not supported by scientific evidence. While vaping is not entirely risk-free, research suggests that it is significantly less harmful than smoking traditional cigarettes and can be an effective smoking cessation aid for some individuals. By debunking common vaping myths and providing accurate information, we can help promote a better understanding of vaping and its potential benefits and risks.

Vaping Regulations and Laws

Vaping Regulations and Laws

In recent years, the vaping industry has experienced rapid growth and innovation, with millions of people worldwide turning to e-cigarettes as an alternative to traditional smoking. However, this surge in popularity has also prompted governments and regulatory agencies to establish laws and regulations to address public health concerns and ensure consumer safety. In this article, we'll explore the current state of vaping regulations and laws, as well as their implications for vapers and the industry as a whole.

Age Restrictions: One of the most fundamental vaping regulations is age restrictions on purchasing and using vaping products. In many countries and regions, including the United States and the European Union, the legal age for purchasing and using vaping products is 18 or 21 years old. These age restrictions are intended to prevent minors from accessing and using vaping products, as nicotine exposure during adolescence can have detrimental effects on brain development and increase the risk of addiction.

Product Standards: Vaping regulations often include standards for the manufacturing, labeling, and packaging of vaping products to ensure their quality, safety, and consistency. These standards may include requirements for product testing, ingredient disclosure, child-resistant packaging, and manufacturing practices. By establishing product standards, regulatory agencies aim to protect consumers from harmful substances and contaminants and promote transparency and accountability within the industry.

Flavor Restrictions: In response to concerns about the appeal of flavored vaping products to young people, some jurisdictions have implemented restrictions on the sale and marketing of flavored e-liquids. These restrictions may prohibit the sale of certain flavors, such as fruit, candy, and dessert flavors, or restrict their availability to adult-only establishments. While flavor restrictions aim to discourage youth vaping, they also raise concerns among adult vapers who rely on flavored e-liquids to quit smoking or reduce harm.

Advertising and Marketing Regulations: Vaping regulations often include restrictions on the advertising and marketing of vaping products to minimize their appeal to minors and prevent misleading or deceptive practices. These regulations may prohibit certain advertising channels, such as television, radio, and print media, and restrict the use of youth-oriented imagery, celebrity endorsements, and health claims in marketing materials. By regulating advertising and marketing, authorities seek to prevent youth initiation, promote public health, and ensure informed consumer decision-making.

Taxation: Some jurisdictions have implemented excise taxes on vaping products to generate revenue and discourage consumption, similar to taxes on traditional tobacco products. These taxes may be based on the volume or nicotine content of vaping products and can significantly increase their cost for consumers. While taxation can generate revenue for public health programs and deter youth vaping, it may also disproportionately impact low-income vapers and hinder access to harm reduction alternatives for smokers.

In conclusion, vaping regulations and laws play a crucial role in shaping the vaping landscape and protecting public health. By establishing age restrictions, product standards, flavor restrictions, advertising regulations, and taxation policies, authorities aim to minimize the potential harms of vaping while maximizing its potential benefits as a smoking cessation aid and harm reduction tool. As the vaping industry continues to evolve, it is essential for policymakers to balance regulatory measures with the needs and preferences of adult vapers and the broader public health goals of reducing smoking-related morbidity and mortality.

Understanding Vaping Regulations and Laws

Understanding Vaping Regulations and Laws

The vaping industry has seen a surge in popularity in recent years, with millions of people worldwide turning to e-cigarettes as an alternative to traditional smoking. However, as the industry continues to grow, governments and regulatory agencies have implemented laws and regulations to address public health concerns and ensure consumer safety. Understanding these regulations and laws is essential for vapers and industry stakeholders alike.

Age Restrictions: One of the most fundamental regulations governing vaping is age restrictions on purchasing and using vaping products. In many countries and regions, including the United States and the European Union, the legal age for purchasing and using vaping products is 18 or 21 years old. These age restrictions aim to prevent minors from accessing and using vaping products, as nicotine exposure during adolescence can have detrimental effects on brain development and increase the risk of addiction.

Product Standards: Vaping regulations often include standards for the manufacturing, labeling, and packaging of vaping products to ensure their quality, safety, and consistency. These standards may require product testing, ingredient disclosure, child-resistant packaging, and adherence to Good Manufacturing Practices (GMP). By establishing product standards, regulatory agencies aim to protect consumers from harmful substances and contaminants and promote transparency and accountability within the industry.

Flavor Restrictions: Concerns about the appeal of flavored vaping products to young people have led to the implementation of flavor restrictions in some jurisdictions. These restrictions may prohibit the sale of certain flavors, such as fruit, candy, and dessert flavors, or restrict their availability to adult-only establishments. While flavor restrictions aim to discourage youth vaping, they also raise concerns among adult vapers who rely on flavored e-liquids to quit smoking or reduce harm.

Advertising and Marketing Regulations: Vaping regulations often include restrictions on the advertising and marketing of vaping products to minimize their appeal to minors and prevent misleading or deceptive practices. These regulations may prohibit certain advertising channels, such as television, radio, and print media, and restrict the use of youth-oriented imagery, celebrity endorsements, and health claims in marketing materials. By regulating advertising and marketing, authorities seek to prevent youth initiation, promote public health, and ensure informed consumer decision-making.

Taxation: Some jurisdictions have implemented excise taxes on vaping products to generate revenue and discourage consumption, similar to taxes on traditional tobacco products. These taxes may be based on the volume or nicotine content of vaping products and can significantly increase their cost for consumers. While taxation can generate revenue for public health programs and deter youth vaping, it may also disproportionately impact low-income vapers and hinder access to harm reduction alternatives for smokers.

In conclusion, understanding vaping regulations and laws is essential for vapers, industry stakeholders, and policymakers alike. By establishing age restrictions, product standards, flavor restrictions, advertising regulations, and taxation policies, authorities aim to minimize the potential harms of vaping while maximizing its potential benefits as a smoking cessation aid and harm reduction tool. As the vaping industry continues to evolve, it is crucial for stakeholders to stay informed about the latest regulatory developments and advocate for policies that balance public health objectives with the needs and preferences of adult vapers.

Have Questions / Comments?

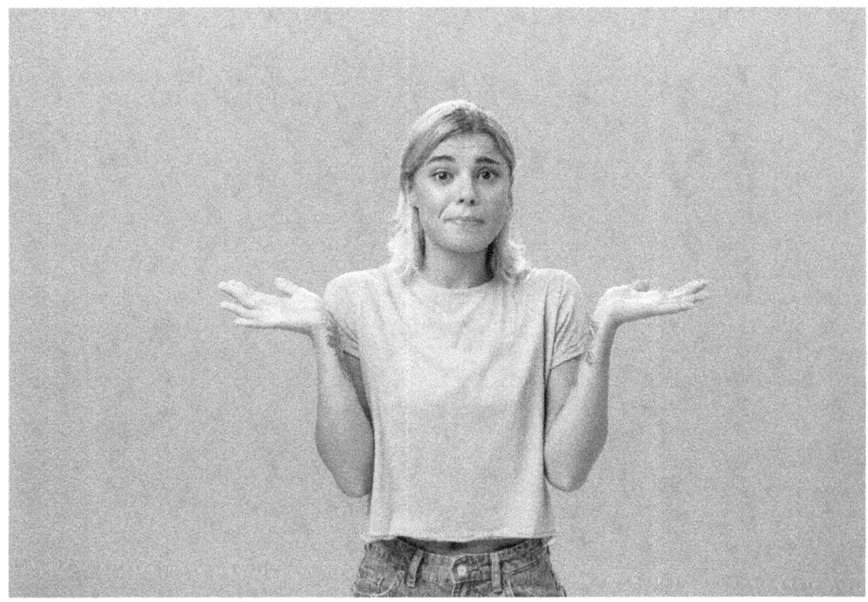

This book was designed to cover as much as possible but I know I have probably missed something, or some new amazing discovery that has just come out.

If you notice something missing or have a question that I failed to answer, please get in touch and let me know. If I can, I will email you an answer and also update the book so others can also benefit from it.

Thanks For Being Awesome :)

Submit Your Questions / Comments At:

https://xspurts.com/posts/questions

Get Another Book Free

We love writing and have produced a huge number of books.

For being one of our amazing readers, we would love to offer you another book we have created, 100% free.

To claim this limited time special offer, simply go to the site below and enter your name and email address.

You will then receive one of my great books, direct to your email account, 100% free!

https://xspurts.com/posts/free-book-offer

www.ingramcontent.com/pod-product-compliance
Lightning Source LLC
Chambersburg PA
CBHW070811260726
48660CB00005B/1811